Healing
*Re*imagined

Reconnecting Traditional Healing *with* Modern Medicine

Karl Ching, DDS

Edited by Jeff Shreve at NY Book Editors
Cover and interior layout by Jasmine Hromjak

Published by Pocket Mole Press

Hardcover: 978-1-7367347-1-1
Softcover: 978-1-7367347-2-8
Ebook: 978-1-7367347-3-5

Disclaimer: Names and identifying details have been changed to protect the privacy of individuals.

First edition published 2021.

ACKNOWLEDGEMENTS

To my parents,
who taught me about life, consciously or otherwise,

To my soul mate and life partner, Karen,
whose love feeds my being,

To my children Everett and Keira,
who graciously allow me to lead their pack,

To my dearest Roy, who taught me forgiveness,
unconditional love, and living in the moment,

To my great aunt and grandmother,
who shepherded me to the trail head,

To my friend and mentor, Stan,
who instantly made me feel like family,

To my San Leandro crew,
the finest group of caring and dedicated professionals,

To all my teachers,
who generously shared their innermost thoughts and lessons,

To each and every indigenous group,
in whose eyes I saw brothers and sisters,

To all the patients with whom I have laughed,
cried, prayed, and commiserated,

To all the readers who have managed to find my writing,
May this book become a vehicle of healing to you, as it was for me.

TABLE OF CONTENTS

PART 3

Establishing and Maintaining Balance

PROLOGUE

As a child, I went through a phase where I would use "why?" as a reply to any question, answer, or statement that was uttered in my general direction. It was partly due to my budding curiosity but probably more so because it annoyed the other person to no end. There was a power in being able to elicit a specific response in virtually anyone. Sometimes, an adult would give me a clear-cut answer and explain the details of how something works, while other times, my questions triggered outright exasperation. In those early days, I was fortunate that several of my conversational counterparts took the time to explain the *whys* and *hows* to many of my questions. Rather than having to beg adults to read me a story, it thrilled me that all these stories came forth just by asking "why?" Nowadays, as a father and answerer of many tens of thousands of questions at home and at work, I am once again reminded of my own perspective as a child.

With much observation and analysis, I developed a keen insight into the wonderful things that we find when we only remember to ask the seemingly magical question. It is with curiosity and pleasant surprise at the replies that come back that I have sought different perspectives into the *whys* that many are afraid to ask (especially with the internally probing ones!). I have been extremely blessed to have not only excellent teachers, but truly genuine caring people that have been willing to reveal to me some of the major lessons of their lives. Traveling the world, I have searched out healers from a multitude of healing traditions only to find striking similarities between widely dispersed groups.

When addressing traditional healing, I am referring specifically to any healing method that has relied on observation, trial, and error over long periods of time, as opposed to the current systematic use of the scientific method developed in the 17th and 18th centuries. Having been primarily educated with the scientific method as a foundation, I also treasure the experiences and lessons learned over lifetimes. Historically, scientific medicine has been pitted diametrically against the traditional medicine that relies more on anecdotal compilations. Many attempts to snuff out traditional medicine rode on the shoulders of religious evangelism throughout the "Age of Discovery" for Europeans. It is no wonder that in North America, indigenous names for places and geographic features have been erased in favor of references to the "devil" and the Christian Bible. However, it was in another era that many traditional modalities suffered their greatest assault: the Scientific Revolution of the 17th century. Efforts to clearly establish the superiority of science over long-held belief systems drove a formidable wedge between the hard-earned wisdom of ancestors and the newest scientific discoveries.

English biologist, anthropologist, and philosopher Thomas Henry Huxley, known for his dogged adherence to Darwin's Theory of Evolution, specifically excluded any mention of morals, ethics, or religious belief systems in his principal address on medical education at the founding of Johns Hopkins School of Medicine.[1] This struggle to gain preeminence may have inadvertently framed progress as a dichotomous zero-sum game. Traditional medicine thus came to be tarnished with the epithets "superstition" and "folklore."

Many generations have been ensnared in this mode of thinking, automatically rejecting long-held traditions. I have come to believe that we have hastily discarded a critical understanding of human nature disguised to appeal to its constituency. In other words, traditional medicine had long understood the power of belief in treatment outcomes and thus tailored the rationale of the treatment to the patient's level of understanding. Rather than dismissing the simplified explanations outright, I sought to further understand the additional undercurrent beyond the obvious trappings. The multilayered complexity of engagement that I found within traditional medicine challenged my ideas of what it means to heal. Simply put, there are multiple levels of interaction, though only one is readily visible to the casual observer.

I am led to the feeling that the colonial mindset—and yes, even cultural chauvinism—of the observers prevented any deeper insight at the time. Indeed, the pleasure derived from achieving a goal is deeply ingrained into our genetics. While it is normal and quite necessary to be proud of your accomplishments, excessive pride consistently blinds one to the equally valid perspectives of others. This pride then becomes an impediment when it impairs the full awareness of other viable possibilities. Only in recent times is the scientific community coming back around to study the significant benefits of traditional healing methods. Even though I am an avid proponent of scientific medicine, the prospect of expanding the horizons of our experiences and abandoning the outdated idea of the zero-sum conflict between science and tradition inspires my optimism.

The tolls of history remain open wounds to many indigenous societies with multiple generations of youth lost to a prevailing culture that dehumanizes, denigrates, and devalues them at every turn. Decimated by genocide and disease, many disparate native groups reeled from these incalculable losses. While many countless indigenous peoples have already lost their cultural and healing traditions, there are flickers of ongoing revival movements to reconnect the wayward groups to other surviving lineages. One example of this desire to preserve the "old ways" is seen in the reclamation of the pipe ceremony in various North American Native tribes. Tribes that had lost their traditions from the passing of their elders were able to reclaim some of the most sacred ceremonies by remembering and borrowing from the revered Oglala Lakota medicine man Black Elk.[2] Another instance is found with the efforts of the Polynesian Voyaging Society, who retraced and revived a disappearing tradition of highly accurate navigation by the stars in the vast Pacific Ocean.[3] It is this race against aging and time that motivates many of the younger generations to preserve their unique cultural identities. These customs that have endured thousands of years now face their most formidable enemy in the imminent aging of the shamans, healers, and elders.

A similar story echoes now in the Amazonian jungles of Peru, Ecuador, Bolivia, and Brazil, as well as the indigenous villages of the Dayak people of Borneo. The elder shamans of the Iban and Bidayuh still serve in their roles but openly express fear for the lack of successors upon their death. The native Sami people of Finland and Norway are experiencing a cultural revival after active government suppression of their culture and language up until the late 1950s.[4] Upon my visit to southern Costa Rica, the Boruca tribe, who had lost much of their healing customs and has no native written language, was actively reconnecting with shaman from the surrounding tribes to retrace their lost heritage. It has become a sacred journey to preserve the native knowledge acquired by generations across thousands of years. When placed alongside the healing modalities that do have a continuous written record, such as Traditional Chinese Medicine and Ayurvedic medicine, there are unexpected commonalities that hint toward our basic needs as human beings.

Traveling extensively and hearing these stories throughout the world, I began to piece together the internal landscape that shapes our very identities. Through personal interaction with various communities that preserve knowledge primarily through oral transmission, I realized that our similarities drew us together ever more tightly as fellow participants in the human experience. The collective wisdom of generations, both simultaneously practical and idealistic, has come to define my own relationships and my manner of communication. I have searched throughout the world for the meaning of healing for decades only to realize that my journey had begun long before I had consciously become aware of it. As a child, my paternal grandmother would often urge me to "take a wider view" whenever I became agitated or deeply upset by an event or situation. As I look back, her wisdom from decades ago now reconnects me to a spectrum of perspectives that seem to resonate from the oldest philosophies. Little did I know that these basic philosophical words were my initiation into finding the meaning of healing. I must profess that only after years of digesting the lessons and sorting my personal observations have I been able to reach a place where I can realistically comprehend and share with my fellow seekers. It is a journey through the indoctrination of schooling, the inherent flexibility of youth, integration of my personal parameters with that of private practice and ultimately reaching a more experienced and—dare I say—wiser philosophical view of the role of healing in our society.

INTRODUCTION

In March of 2019, a hospital in Fremont, California first used a video-link robot to inform relatives that their 78-year-old patient and family patriarch was dying and there was no treatment that was going to improve his situation. The treating physician was unavailable to deliver the news, so an off-site doctor quickly read the computerized treatment notes and sat for the video-call. The robot with video-link monitor then rolled up to the unsuspecting family and initiated the conversation. Despite the hospital protocol calling for another nurse or doctor to be present in the consultation room during this communication, this second person never made the meeting. The lone replacement physician, who had not been directly involved with the patient's treatment, proceeded to deliver a "matter-of-fact" statement regarding the poor prognosis. The already anxious family was so shocked and distraught by the absence of empathy, compassion and connection, they were literally speechless. The result was a monumental failure of humanistic communication.

In this single episode, many of our greatest fears about the possible future of medicine were realized. In a moment when connection and empathy were most necessary, the bad news was delivered through a robot with a computer monitor, a cold detached piece of machinery on wheels. What was it about the presentation that compounded the injury to a person already facing their impending death? For the managing corporate entity of the hospital, it was perhaps not their finest day in implementing new technology. To the patient and his family, it was nothing short of devastating, humiliating, and dehumanizing. Was this truly the future that medicine had in mind for us?

Like all healthcare practitioners, we are subject to the changing characteristics of our professions both from a societal standpoint, as well as the
business realities. Today, many new medical and dental school graduates are
finding employment not in the small private practices of old but as employees of either large group practices or medical corporations that dictate the
business parameters of their everyday practice. This trend was apparent in
the medical community for many years,[5] and has migrated to the dental
community with much of the same effects. Amidst these changes, the
unspoken skills that had heretofore been transferred from an older more
experienced practitioner to a young impressionable associate over years are
now left without a venue. Without the classroom of private practice, we are
losing the conditions under which these subtle skills can naturally develop.
While scientific medicine has drawn a strong distinction between technical expertise and compassion, I am not alone in my belief that social and
empathic skills should be additional criteria for competency.[6]

In my years as a periodontist, I've noticed an inclination of patients
to avoid and ignore necessary treatment. There are few negative motivators as powerful as pain and expense. For those who are unfamiliar
with periodontics, it is a Board-recognized specialty of dentistry which
specializes in gum disease diagnosis and treatment, dental implant place-
ment and preparation, as well as hard and soft tissue regeneration. It is
a specialty that has traditionally been by referral (although the current
industry trends do include a primary care option) and is often dreaded
by patients. As one such periodontist who is aware of these sensitivities, I
found it extremely important to improve patient experiences by making
it less traumatic and more friendly.

I have witnessed fear for my entire dental career and find that the
emotional response to surgery, especially dental surgery, can be as debilitating as the physical illness itself. We must acknowledge that physical
healing does not address the emotional damage inflicted in the process of
realizing our own mortality.

I must state that many of the ideas presented here may be very familiar to various experts in their field, and I am deeply indebted to them for their ingenuity and acumen in the understanding of human nature. It is in the milieu of ideas that pass through my personal lens that I share my combination of experiences in the hope that it may enhance the patient experience and raise the watermark for medical care in all its forms. I have been fortunate to practice in an environment that has allowed prolonged observations on a wide spectrum of patient responses to treatment. What caused patients to respond to the potential of impending pain with varying levels of resolve? How does the approach of the healthcare practitioner encourage acceptance and long-term compliance? In this case, it is the context and application of these ideas that is novel. There is much to be learned when asking the simple question, "What just happened here?"

It is my sincere hope that this discourse will improve the level of communication between the doctor or healthcare worker and the patient so that our approach will address not only medicine on the physical level but also encompass the complete emotional restoration of the patient. There is little doubt that modern medicine excels at treating acute trauma. However, in disorders of long-term breakdown, traditional healing still has much to offer. A day may dawn when the physical trauma of treatment is reduced to an afterthought. Nevertheless, the importance of treating a patient as a whole cannot be understated.

From my experience, the impression of quality in medicine has been heavily reliant on a list of past training locations and titles achieved. This in turn has proven an unreliable indicator of whether a doctor can effectively connect with their patients and raise the overall health of their community.

Imagine instead, a medical and dental world in which an effective healing approach could be taught and implemented on a wide scale, especially on the community level and on the front lines. I am not proposing to teach a preset personality with a canned, one-size-fits-all understanding.

My hope is that we may accept myriad lessons from traditional medicine that have served humanity for thousands of years and forge a more comprehensive idea of healing. This both new and old method of approaching a new patient will help doctors and patients alike engage with each other in a more detailed and systematic way. Perhaps we can create a critical mass of desire to raise the overall quality of patient care to a level commensurate with all the wonderful technological advances in the modern medical world.

As a trained dentist and surgeon, I spent a significant amount of time seeking technical expertise and knowledge, but I found that this path to learning the art and science leads to a significant limitation. There is always the challenge of communicating knowledge to a patient, presenting all the known benefits and disadvantages. Often much is lost in the translation and application of knowledge into a diagnosis, description of treatment options, and creation of a workable and agreeable treatment plan. In other words, the level of communication between the healthcare worker and the patient has been and is still a significant bottleneck to the necessary end point of quality medical care. Fluent communication may appear to be a matter of linguistics and diction, but there is the matter of what is *said* versus what is *meant*, which oftentimes complicates the already stressful situation of seeking medical care. The multitude of backgrounds, cultures, and languages of the patients that seek our care further increase the complexity of our need to rapidly grasp the pure intent of the visit. At various times, the healthcare practitioner must fill the roles of confidante, counselor, doctor, and friend.

The term *bedside manner* encompasses the ability to smoothly navigate the intricacies of managing the diagnosis, informing the patient, addressing the questions and concerns with the options, and managing expectations involved with the treatment.

In order to treat a patient completely, it is imperative that the timing at which each role becomes preeminent be dictated by the communicated message from the patient. Communication between healthcare worker and patient must be clear and precise for the doctor to accurately assess the disorder. However, we have all experienced the situation when people don't say what they truly mean. To paraphrase the famous Greek physician Galen: do not always listen to what a patient is saying (verbally) but observe carefully and see with your own eyes to develop your diagnosis.

The immediate question that comes to mind is: How do we see what a patient really means? Clearly, putting yourself into the perspective of the patient requires a bird's eye view of the psychological dynamics at play.

The scope of our current discussion does not include the technical aspects of how to perform any particular procedure. Rather, we elevate the importance of the details in leading a patient from one aspect to the next with clear and comforting communication that inspires confidence. The details in *how* you are able to manage the situation contributes significantly to the healing process in addition to *what* you directly said to the patient. This includes many aspects of communication that *show* your caring and careful guidance in addition to the hard facts that you *tell* them. In understanding the basics of the universal aspects of human communication, we may yet have a chance to improve our soft skills systematically. We live in a society that emphasizes choice in medical treatments, and we as healthcare workers must accept that patients do make the ultimate decision to either stay in our care or seek other options.

There is always the concern of cost-benefit ratio in every consideration of a possible treatment plan. Sometimes, there just is not a very good option at the time. Whatever I have learned and trained for years to do may or may not be a palatable solution to patients based on their perspective. There are few things as upsetting as spending hours and weeks on a project, getting the desired result, and then realizing that the patient is less than thrilled with the outcome. Alas, I came upon my only clear understanding, which is that there is much more to this practice of healing than the hard/technical skills.

Throughout my travels, I have expressed a special interest in the healing traditions of indigenous cultures. While some patients and their healers came from the same communities and cultures, others were Western patients desperately seeking a solution to medical or psychiatric issues that defied modern medicine. Consistently I witnessed interviews, ceremonies, and use of medicinal herbs that helped unravel the circumstances that led to the illnesses. They also drew the patients into rich and varied belief systems that clearly reflected the values and experiences of the healer's particular culture. All of the people and places that I visited and who so graciously shared their ancestral knowledge had an ultimate goal in mind for all of their patients. Each and every one sought *balance* as the goal of their treatments.

This book is organized into three main sections: 1) Expanding Awareness, 2) Cultivating Belief, and 3) Establishing and Maintaining Balance. Part One deals with extending all of our senses to include the verbal communications and expressions as well as the tacit non-spoken communications that are often overlooked. These include, but are not limited to body language, assessment of feelings, and patterns of personality imbalances. This awareness of both verbal and non-verbal communication is key to gleaning more information in a short period of time, helping us build the context around a patient's medical problem/s. Part Two examines the mental building blocks that evolve into trust and belief in our everyday interactions. Modern medicine has only begun to explore the significant improvements in healing when fully engaging a patient's belief systems. Part Three discusses how we can balance a number of parameters to attain a more harmonious state that may be more conducive to long-term healing.

As I incorporated the essence of my interactions with traditional healing methods throughout our world, these three commonalities surfaced and resurfaced time and again. Despite the vast differences in environments under which the source groups evolved, the universality of these lessons struck me as fundamental to the human condition. From the Arctic regions to the islands of the South Pacific, the genial smiles and kind words that greeted me from diverse indigenous groups converge into a mutual need in healing that reaches into our very identities and consciousnesses.

PART 1

Expanding Awareness

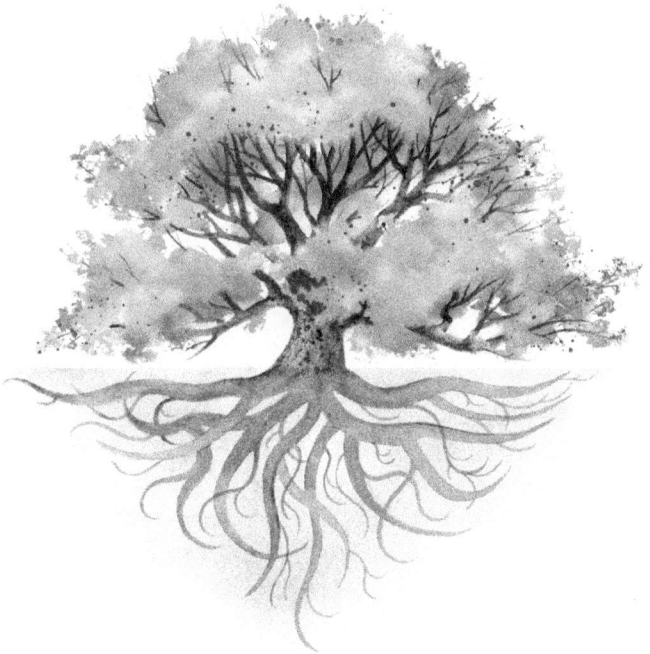

Awareness, a term that encompasses not only knowing something but also being conscious, feeling, and cognitively poised to respond—with full attention, functionally engaged, yet holding back, waiting for the right moment to act. It includes careful observation, recognition of the current situation, and imminent formulation of a plan of attack. In this manner, it is both an active and passive word that initiates our journey towards healing.

We begin with a traditional medicine that is familiar to most western trained healthcare practitioners, as there is abundant detailed historical documentation. The medicine of Classical Greece indeed fits squarely into our definition of traditional medicine in that it is rich in observation, trial and error, and built upon generations of knowledge. The Hippocratic Oath, taken by medical students upon graduation, echoes back to the ethical standards set forth by the physician Hippocrates of Kos. His legacy was the establishment of medicine as an independent discipline that branched off from philosophy and theology.

In the second century CE, in Rome, Greece, and Turkey, Aelius Galenus, more commonly known as Galen of Pergamon, not only built upon the works of Hippocrates but became the single most influential Western physician for the next 1300 years by seeking to expand his awareness of the mammalian body and its supporting systems.[7] Since the dissection of the human body was outlawed by Roman law since approximately 150 BCE, he spent years dissecting first monkeys, then pigs, cattle, and sheep to divulge the inner workings of their anatomies. Traveling widely and learning from the preeminent teachers and philosophers of the day, he returned to his hometown Pergamon at the age of 28 to tend to the health of gladiators. In studying their wounds, he was able to develop his surgical techniques and an unparalleled (at the time) knowledge of trauma medicine. After five years he brought his knowledge and techniques to Rome, where he firmly established his skills to none other than Marcus Aurelius, emperor of Rome. To his patients as well as his students, Galen possessed a knowledge and awareness of medicine that seemed almost supernatural.

In walking among the ruins of Pergamon in modern-day Turkey, we can easily imagine Galen's observations as early advances in science, yet we must make a clear distinction between awareness and science. Awareness is a personal experience in finding knowledge by way of the senses and including observation, testing, and verification. Science is a systematic method of finding knowledge through proposal of a hypothesis, testing, and then either acceptance or rejection of the hypothesis. While awareness can include knowledge learned from the scientific method, science does not always explain the wide range of awareness of the human experience. Another way of saying it is simply that *awareness* is a wider term that includes science but encompasses other aspects that have been experienced but not yet systematically studied. In a sense, we as a culture have a limited sense of personal involvement in the acquisition of knowledge, as it has been outsourced to scientists.

How many people can you account for who are highly effective at learning from a book or the internet, yet cannot practically apply what they have memorized? The recognition, adaptation, improvisation, and application of knowledge that is intrinsic to outstanding awareness is not automatically built in to a spoon-fed education. Awareness requires a personal attention to the subject at hand that cannot be limited to book learning. Many healthcare practitioners rely heavily on lab tests to rule out possibilities when those same lab tests should be tools to confirm what they already know. It is no coincidence that both traditional Greek as well as Chinese medicine include (but are not limited to) visual, facial, tongue, pulse, percussion, palpation, sound, smell, and excretion examinations. Essentially, they employ all the senses of the human body to detect illness.

It is this very awareness that allows us to gather information about our surroundings and the people around us. This may include any tidbit of relevant knowledge that helps us improve our understanding of any given scenario. Expanding our awareness to encompass that of ourselves and our patients enables us to compare and contrast their situations with known models of health. The careful examination not only gives us an opportunity to collect pertinent details, but also demonstrates an outward display of thoroughness to the patient.

Combined with our respective medical training, we can take the information gathered and incrementally piece together the story of any illness. This insight is essential to the assessment of any physical or mental ailment. When we fully evaluate the information gathered, we begin to see patterns and recognize signs of future risk. It is then that we begin to deal in projections and probabilities of future illness due to current trajectories, i.e., relationships between cholesterol levels and future heart disease. This would have been deemed as uncommon foresight in centuries past. However, it is now clearly in the realm of modern medicine to employ this foresight to allow longer-term solutions that will not only cure the illness but establish the adaptations necessary to prevent relapse and minimize built-in susceptibilities.

Let us consider the archetype of a patient that arrives in our care (assuming it is not an acute emergency) who simply states that she wants "to smile again." Many healthcare practitioners have seen this person, and we have seen her in many different forms and sizes. For our purposes, let us call her Ella.

This seemingly simple statement of wanting to smile again can be an extremely loaded one, especially if we consider the many angles from which we can read it. Depending on the branch of medicine/healing from which we are approaching, this can equate to a statement on mental health, family responsibilities, love life, depression, functional or esthetic dental problems, physical cosmetic surgery imperfections, or really any type of personal dissatisfactions.

It is from this point that we begin our journey into filling in the circumstances around the statement of wanting to smile again. Indeed, our challenge is to reveal the reasons for Ella's dissatisfaction to the physical action that finally presents to us. Through conversation, observation, examination, and extrapolation of information, we can track and trace the thread of this statement through the context of her life. With each piece of information that we compile on Ella, we can fill in the spaces to create a profile that helps us fully understand her viewpoint. As such, we begin with the part of the initial consultation that is yet to be covered in conventional training.

CHAPTER 1

Making Observation Your Superpower

A natural starting point of any discussion of the patient-doctor relationship is the initial contact at the first appointment. It is usually this potentially awkward meeting that allows a healthcare practitioner to learn more about a patient's chief complaint and background. It is also a chance for the patient to gauge their comfort level and expectations with the practitioner. I have often found the initial consultation to be one of the more taxing types of appointments. There are usually many expectations that are unspoken, yet we have very little time to discern the entire context of the patient's problem. How we approach the patient clearly has a way of determining what information they choose to reveal. These variations in approach have been coined *bedside manner* and has been described as "a way with words," or positive "personality traits" that defy common categorization. Life experience and charisma, which could not be determined on paper, certainly contribute to this ability to connect. However, you almost need to see the doctor in their element interacting with patients to tell if they have the magic touch. In fact, these personality traits can either improve or worsen a miscommunication to the point of initiating legal proceedings.

For us to venture further into our discussion, we must first peer backwards into the historical record. *Bedside manner* is an umbrella term that incorporates a combination of effective communication, mannerisms, ethics, decorum, etiquette, empathy, as well as character. We can trace the current lineage and understanding of the term from Hippocrates in fourth century BCE Greece. Barry Silverman, MD,[8] provided an elegant overview of the history of physician behavior and bedside manner centering on the origins of the western tradition in Greek times and following into the evolution of the American viewpoint from the nineteenth to twentieth centuries. Peculiarly, we owe our current expectations of the bedside manner of a modern physician to the era in which it rapidly spread around the world. With the historical expansion of the British Empire, the credibility of scientific medicine rode on the back of the military science which allowed conquest of large swaths of the globe. As a result, many of our ideas on proper behavior for healthcare practitioners have roots in antiquated ideas of the Victorian gentleman and the paternalistic (some might say patronizing) notion of *noblesse oblige*.

Traditional healing, on the other hand, is practiced more on the local level within communities where the healer and patient were better acquainted. This bond formed by common culture and history allows a much richer understanding of a patient's social background. By and large, these traditional healers spend a greater amount of time interviewing the patient and working through the entire history of the illness. As such, the context of the illness in a patient's life is more easily discerned compared to modern medicine. While there may still be country doctors in small towns stateside practicing their noble professions, there is a decreasing opportunity for newer generations of doctors and healthcare workers to develop their craft under proper guidance.

So, we will examine the process to reconstruct the context of any patient from externally discernible criteria (verbal communication and body language) and work our way towards the internal aspects (psychology and neurology). Upon initiation of verbal communication, healthcare practitioners will not only need to take note of the literal meanings of the conversation but establish the context in which those words are delivered. The specific choice of words and diction should be carefully considered. This tends to be the most easily accessible portion of the information-gathering process, as we can take a record of the specific words used and review them as needed. When establishing the context, one major aim is to discover the "normal" baseline for the patient. In other words, does the patient's idea of normal match the societal and medical idea of normal? Often times, some patients may have been coping with chronic pain and have adapted to a high level of discomfort. For them, regular use of excessive amounts of painkillers may be "normal."

While it may seem simplistic to say that words convey meaning, there is deeper significance when dealing with patients who may or may not be withholding pertinent information both consciously and subconsciously. The choice of words may even be considered negative, evasive, affirmative, or mildly agreeable (but not quite effusive). In our well-developed market economy, most people are considered potential customers by a vast number and variety of consumer companies. The public is already so well conditioned to someone trying to sell them something. As patients, they bring that stance with them into their initial appointments despite the change in environment. Yet, we cannot deny that there is a component of healthcare that is retail oriented and elective in nature.

Regardless of your personality, the greater the social exchange during that initial two-to-five-minute period of meeting a patient, the greater the amount of data you have to establish the patient's context. We can certainly obtain the standard chief complaint and take a medical history while keeping one eye on any visible signs of disease, discomfort, and distress.

On top of assessing the technical needs of a patient, there must be an accurate estimation of the unspoken aspects. When listening to how a person makes a statement, our senses will require finer tuning. What are the feelings involved when a person speaks? Are the words spoken with humor, sarcasm, pain, anger, exasperation, or annoyance? When a patient starts with a short statement, "On my last physical, my doctor told me I have a gum infection," do we hear only what is explicitly said? Can we also surmise that what they excluded may also be important to our treatment? What do they mean by the phrase *my doctor told me*? Is there a hint of annoyance, since their diagnosis seems to be a greater concern for the doctor than it is for him/her? We can also hear from this statement that there is no mention of active pain. The unspoken part of this consultation may give clues as to the range of expectations that are anticipated but not always articulated for convenient consumption.

Much of the internal dialogue within my mind involves opening up vaguely described senses that combine verbal cues with body language and placing them within a context of a patient's background (ethnic, economic, age, gender, etc.). Opening up these senses requires a great deal of concentration and active awareness. At the same time we must pay attention to the subtle cues of the subconscious mind.

Our conscious minds can handle a limited number of items before it is overwhelmed. The subconscious mind, however, can keep track of many thousands of feedback indicators that dictate our homeostasis and overall well-being. While we can usually handle five to nine windows[9] simultaneously open on our computers, our subconscious minds can track the balance of hundreds of muscles along with the thousands of innervations that allow the seemingly simple act of walking or running.

What may seem to be a gut feeling or intuition may actually be a message from your subconscious mind. Have you ever had a deep suspicion about something but were unable to prove it, and then later found out that your inner voice was strikingly accurate? Rather than looking at it from a paranormal perspective, consider that gut feeling to be a direct communication from your subconscious mind. Essentially, each of our five senses gives us vast amounts of information which we collect as memory.

Information deemed important is communicated back to the conscious mind for action. As our language abilities are not processed through the subconscious, this part of the mind is left with communicating through pictures, sounds, smells, tastes, touch, and feelings. Some may refer to these feelings as intuition. Whatever you choose to call it, discounting the communication would be an oversight.

Once we gather enough information to develop an understanding of the context of the patient's original statement, we can begin to identify the urgency of this chief complaint as it is seen through the patient's eyes. This context may reveal that the problem is a regularly recurring one, as opposed to being a beginning sign of disease. We may also discover that their presented problem is secondary to a systemic immune suppression from another health challenge.

As we begin to piece together the information presented to us, a greater picture reveals itself, and we can then direct further questioning to establish the overall health status of our patient.

CHAPTER 2

Reading
Body Language

O ne of the key elements of assessing patient disposition will be verbal communication. However, even more can be ascertained through reading body language. We can define *body language* as the process of communicating nonverbally through conscious or unconscious gestures and movements. Body language is often the most reliable indicator of a person's subconscious disposition. The patient may or may not be aware of how they present their body language, yet it can be most revealing of their current state of well-being. Some estimates place the amount of communication conveyed non-verbally at 60-65%.[10] Most of us can already read many of the emotions possible as it is a significant part of growing up in our culture. Still, a careful examination of this subject may yield variations in different cultures globally.

The awareness of this aspect of bedside manner will hopefully allow us to understand that verbal communication can be placed into a context of overall communication. When the verbal and non-verbal messages match, we can confirm that the communicated message is received. However, when they do not match, we may need to seek clarification, or we may have reason to suspect an ulterior motive or agenda. When we are initially learning to read baseline emotions, much can be gleaned through careful observation of animals and young children, especially household pets, infants, and children immediately prior to proper language development. There is fortunately a rich environment into which we can all delve into for the purpose of honing our awareness skills. Once again, there will be significant differences in the body language of different cultures, and distinctions are necessary between the culture of upbringing versus the common culture of business and daily public interaction.

In modern psychology, J.A. Fodor[11] had revisited the idea of specific sections of the brain devoted to particular functions. He called his theory Modularity of the Mind, which attempted to explain the cognition necessary from initial sensory input (sight, sound, smell, touch, taste) into pathways that compute into actionable information. In other words, combinations of senses trigger a reflex translation into meaningful data. This data is then categorized, and the mind selects a "module" that most likely allows the individual to best adapt to the situation at hand.

In 2013, psychologists Douglas Kenrick and Vladas Griskevicius[12] further elaborated on this subject by identifying seven modules that affect everyday behavior: 1) Self-Protection, 2) Mate Attraction, 3) Mate Retention, 4) Affiliation (friendships, alliances, etc.), 5) Kin Care (taking care of family), 6) Status, and 7) Disease Avoidance. While there is not yet unanimous agreement on the number and content of modules, these categories represent the expectations that a person's mind holds when walking into a situation.

Stated another way, these modules are default programs specifically encoded into our genetics. Your brain takes sensory information and shifts your stance into the best mode (or module) that will put you in position to face the upcoming challenge. One possible analogy would involve a driver sensing a rocky road ahead and switching from 2-wheel drive to 4-wheel drive mode. Preparing for a rougher ride, the driver may grip the steering wheel tighter, and sit up for a better view as well. With this psychological model of modularity in mind, consider the body language of each module. While there are variances between individuals, there seems to be a tremendous consistency in the level of openness of our stance based on the currently selected module.

Overall body language can be categorized into spinal posture, eye contact, facial expressions, and expressions with the limbs. The spinal posture can refer to head position in relation to the person with which you are conversing, shoulder direction, degree of opening of the shoulders, and direction of the hips. In western culture, a direct communication approach is seen as honest and straightforward.

In general, the body language displays anywhere on a spectrum from entirely closed posture, seen in Disease Avoidance, to completely open in Mate Attraction. The Self-Protection module typically displays a closed posture, but with additional eye contact and facial expressions of warning. In this module, a person senses a potentially dangerous environment and the subconscious increases the heart rate, releases adrenaline (also called epinephrine), dilates the pupils of the eyes for better vision, and prepares for either fight or flight. Mate Retention, Affiliation, and Kin Care will be more on the open posture side of the spectrum, with variations in intimacy. For Status, we may see more of an open posture, but with an underlying strength that projects confidence and power. While the outward appearance could be a false projection, the underlying truth is not as important when jockeying for status.

Spinal Posture

The head position is considered open and neutral if the eyes and chin are level with their conversational partner. A chin held high can be interpreted as excessive pride, and one held low can be seen as low self-esteem, or possibly having something to hide. As such, a straight spine, shoulders and hips directly facing the person with whom they are talking, relaxed open shoulders leading to ease of breathing, are considered a strong neutral and honest position from which to speak. These positions indicate that there is no surprise and no ulterior motive behind the communication. The shoulder position can be open (shoulders held to open the ribcage for breathing) or slouched forward, which impairs the breath. Hips facing the other person are also aimed at facilitating a direct connection. Any positioning of the posture that deviates from a direct connection can be read as an impaired or partial communication. A spinal posture held upright and straight is a sign of confidence, and willingness to directly engage in communication. This open posture outwardly displays a friendly, open, and engaging demeanor.

A person turned to the side with their shoulders and hips as they are speaking may indicate that they are not fully engaged in communication with you and may be impatient to go elsewhere. This closed posture expresses disagreement, hostility, and a hint of anxiety. There are many reasons for an unwillingness to fully engage, and the variety of interpretations are too numerous to cite. The main idea to take away is that every person can present as a puzzle, and when you reach a point where you can share a perspective together, you have made a worthwhile connection.

Eye Contact

The eyes are considered "the window to the soul" for good reason. Much can be gleaned from the willingness of a person to engage in a conversation with direct eye contact. The idea that someone can look into your eyes and see your thoughts is a widespread belief, despite not having much evidence to prove it. Constant and/or intermittent averted eye contact, frequent blinking, and looking at the ceiling or floor can certainly make a conversation awkward. If this persists beyond the initiation of the conversation, there is reason to believe that the person has alternative plans or something to hide, or your communication is failing. Discomfort, anxiety, and distraction are but a few of the reasons for the disturbance in firm connection through the eyes. On the other hand, prolonged staring may be construed as threatening. A wide opening of the eyes and arching of the eyebrows may show surprise or exasperation.

Facial Expressions

Facial expressions can convey a tremendous amount of information without ever resorting to speech. Imagine the multitudes of emojis and facial expressions for the basic emotions of happiness, sadness, anger, fear, confusion, just to name a few. You may have a person verbally tell you one thing and have their facial expressions betray their true feelings. Much can be read from the tension in the facial muscles, especially the eyebrows and the muscles around the mouth.

When researchers studied the domestication of dogs, they found a profound adaptation in the muscles of the eyes of wild dogs which were not present in wolves. The eye muscles of the eyebrows allowed the dogs to enhance their show of emotion and simulated the look of a child (paedomorphism) which elicited a physical response in humans.[13] This response is directly measured in the release of the hormone oxytocin (hormone that triggers a nurturing response) in human brains and may have resulted in the close relationship between humans and canines. Evidence has shown that oxytocin triggers a release of dopamine (we will explain further in Chapter 5) in the ventral tegmental area of the brain.[14]

The muscles around the mouth also tend to reveal much about a person's feelings. Of course, a smile is universally seen as a friendly gesture, but the context of a smile may also be used to show sarcasm, cynicism, and aggression. Frowns and grimacing in general are negative signs indicative of unhappiness, anger, or sadness. Biting one's lip typically reveals tension, anxiety, and insecurity, while pursing of the lips (tensing the muscles around the mouth) is a firm display of disapproval. Some of these facial expressions may cross species boundaries as well. Luckily, many facial expressions cross cultural boundaries and show remarkable similarity across the world.

Expressions with the Hands, Arms, and Legs

Expression with the limbs refers to the use of hands, arms, and leg movements. Crossing the arms and/or legs often indicate that the person is feeling defensive, withdrawing from attention, and closed off to new ideas. Cracking knuckles, tapping fingers, or other types of fidgeting show a nervous energy that can signal anxiety, boredom, impatience, or frustration. Hands on the hips may be a sign of being ready and poised to start, as well as being in control and mild aggression. Any covering of the face with the hands or holding the chin and mouth reveals an attempt to conceal or repress an emotion, as well as a reconsideration of an idea. Feet facing the exit to a room has also been associated with impatience, frustration, or a general feeling of wanting to leave.

The Body Language of Positive Emotions

Happiness, joy, and hopefulness are relatively easy emotions to spot as a person smiles, shoulders are open, the breathing is deeper and unlabored, their energy level becomes animated, and often they cannot sit still. Positive emotions stem from the freedom and creativity of initial actions and can be spontaneous in nature. They represent the wonder of discovery in the eyes of children and the delight in exploring new and possibly wonderful things that stimulate and intrigue the conscious mind. The eyes are a large part of the body language here, as a smile can reach into the periorbital (around the eyes) area. The eyebrows are level-to-arched in the center when in the positive emotive mode. There is a general relaxed atmosphere where pressure to do something or to be a certain way is not felt. The individual is fully capable of carrying the weight of what is asked of them. This body language can be placed within the context of playfulness, joking, and/or outwardly seeking connections. There is an overall feeling of capability of doing anything that comes to mind. This generally gives a feeling of power over one's own destiny, and of "Yes, I can." This positive energy is unmistakable and will help you spot when a previously unbalanced point is brought back into balance. This should be a baseline for assessing a healthy steady state.

The Body Language of Nervousness and Indecision

A frequently seen issue is with patients who are not able to make decisions and exhibit a nervous fidgety demeanor. Nervous people may exhibit rather erratic bodily movements, clenching of muscles in the hand and face, or excessive sweating from the head, neck, back, armpits, as well as the hands and feet. There is an inherent discomfort in making the wrong choice and relating these choices to their own sense of self-worth. These small nervous movements, as well as pacing and repeatedly standing up and sitting down, may be seen as a translation of internal indecision and nervous energy into physical movement. Eyes may dart in different directions with quick rapid movements. Imagine the movements of a squirrel darting across a road and changing directions multiple times as it crosses.

Rather than being weak, as much of our society deems the nervous person, the reality is that many people exhibiting these qualities can intellectually see the distinct benefits of many different situations. They are often not able to make a quick snap decision because of information overload from considering the possible advantages of each perspective. This heightened intellectual capability allows them to sort through much of what they perceive. Yet, they are also exceptionally aware of the implications placed upon them by society for what appears to be indecisiveness. The stakes of making a "poor" choice are dramatically increased as they are subject to the judgment from both themselves, their loved ones, and their social circles.

This inherent criticism from a societal standpoint places tremendous pressure for nervous individuals to make faster decisions lest they fulfill the stereotype of a bungling fool. However, the faster the decision is made, the less time there is to sort out all the advantages and disadvantages. This becomes a negative cycle that forces the individual repeatedly into a situation where they are at their worst and most unable to utilize their gifts of intelligence and observation to their advantage. There is simply less and less time to sort through all the possible outcomes prior to committing to a course of action. It is much of this criticism that the nervous individual is particularly sensitive to, thus making for a self-perpetuating cycle of increasing pressure to make quicker decisions and never enough time to sort through too much information.

The inherent nature of a nervous patient compromises their own view of their abilities to empower themselves for any given task. Thus, they are clearly distinguished from others based on their diminished capability. This self-judgment is critical in continuing this cycle of indecision and ultimately despair. In many ways, the mere anticipation of having to decide becomes an ordeal which echoes the traumas of many past negative experiences in decision-making. This is not unlike a post-traumatic stress disorder but applied to a daily necessity such as deciding whether you want coffee or tea.

The Body Language of Negative Emotions: Fear and Pain

When we target the healing environment, we will need to have a baseline for assessing the emotions. For patients that step into our office, it begins with something as simple as reading pain. One major pillar of negative emotions is pain, and the resulting suffering is both physical and emotional. We can all imagine the grimace on the face with clenching and grinding of teeth, sweating, bulging veins, and facial flushing indicating increased blood flow to the face. Examining further down the body from the head leads us to shoulders and neck holding tension, sometimes with activation of the neck muscles from the jaw all the way down to the collarbone. We often see the platysma muscle (the thin sheet of muscle covering the jawline down to the collarbone) on the front of the neck straining as a result of clenching of the teeth. Flexing of the fingers and forearms are also not to be neglected. You can imagine the common scene of a patient in a dental chair gripping the armrest tightly until the skin on their hands and fingers blanches. The breathing is often shallow and quick. Unintentional constriction of the muscles of the arms, hands, legs, and or an overall agitated demeanor will indicate active pain.

Fear is another pillar of negative emotion and is more reactionary in nature. Typically, a fear develops after a negative consequence from an action. Let's say, for example, we have a child who is learning how to ride a bicycle. She scoots along seated on the saddle with both feet off the floor and feels the feeling of the wind in her face and hair. She overcompensates for a turn and instantly lands on her leg and outstretched hand with scuffs in her skin and some bleeding. Feeling the searing pain in the skin of her hand and leg, she lets out a shriek. After the shock of the fall and the pain in her hand and leg starts to wane, she may not be as eager to get back on the bicycle. The longer this episode replays in her mind, the stronger the fear of getting back onto the bike. This fear is a natural response that activates learning in the brain to avoid a similar negative consequence. Somehow the surest way to avoid the pain of falling is to not ride a bicycle at all.

The body language of fear clearly displays a penchant for concealment and avoidance of eye contact. There is a downward angle to the head that shows deference and submission. The shoulders are often slumped and turned to the side to avoid confrontation. The hands and feet are subdued and usually at the side or placed directly in front of the lap to show a lack of threat.

From an emotional standpoint, the anticipation of the impending pain is sometimes more agonizing than the actual pain itself. The aforementioned body language will be seen in a person who is awaiting something that they are convinced will be painful. You may see that over time, the negative effect on a person grows despite the ultimate pain being the same. The mind amplifies the impending pain as the healing from the first episode had not yet completed. Thus, every subsequent episode of pain relives the previous cases and the current case simultaneously. Case in point: There are many children that do not cry when given their first injection. Over time with multiple injections, how they decide to accept the idea of having to get an injection will ultimately determine whether they accept the pain as a necessary part of the treatment. Conversely, the repeated replay of this initial pain in their minds turn it into something much greater. We can see that it is in the response that these phobias develop. The power of the mind is indeed immense that we can convince ourselves that nothing could be worse than a particular type of pain.

Chronic pain presents itself with some differences in that the body has had some time to adapt. There is an emotional aspect to chronic pain that can include all the previously mentioned active pain symptoms but also include a resigned feeling of defeat. Slumping shoulders, sagging eyelids, dark circles under the eyes, and/or an overall tired, beat down disposition can certainly tell much about the emotional state of a patient. Many of the facial muscles of mastication (chewing muscles) are a clear indicator of underlying stress. The facial emotive muscles of the eyebrows, cheeks, and forehead are additional indications of stress.

For example, a furrow between the eyebrows shows frequent squinting which can connote a skepticism or a concerned look. Breathing is deep and labored with long sighs and measured expirations. A more detailed examination may reveal wrinkle lines that show a history of frequent muscle innervation and contraction.

The speed of movement will also give an indication as to the active or passive nature of pain. Active pain is usually represented by quicker muscle movement, as the body and psyche has not been subject to a prolonged struggle, so to speak. When the sense of pain is prolonged, we can see the cumulative fatigue that adds to the perceived burden on top of normal everyday function. This results in slower, more labored muscle movements in general. Over the course of time, such chronic conditions can lead to a feeling of defeat and depression. Chronic pain can lead to a very isolating feeling when nobody else truly feels your pain and there is no quick nor convenient way of resolving it. Thus, depression and loneliness come hand in hand, and has been associated with various forms of self-treatment involving pain reliever medications.

Recently, more attention has been brought to depression and other types of psychological imbalances. The body language of depression is very similar to that of chronic pain but can be more subtle, as the person has had a chance to adapt longer and sometimes can even mask the symptoms. There are obvious signs of negativity, such as sloping shoulders, slower movements, facial signs of fatigue. The eyes have a way of expressing emptiness and resignation to a given fate. We may need to combine these observations with the context provided in verbal questioning.

Powerlessness is particularly noteworthy as a sign of the onset of depression. One of the clearer signs of depression is resignation to a negative fate. I've often heard the lament "I always get the shaft" or "we always get screwed." We may be able to see that the patient constantly revisits the idea that the most negative outcome is the most likely outcome. This self-programming of the negative outcome is a difficult cycle to escape, as it may become self-fulfilling. When we begin to envision our own inability with all the associated details of failure, how much are we planning our own negative outcome? We must also consider the societal pressures on those who carry a negative outlook. The judgment of their ability to exist as a productive member of a family, a profession, or society itself weighs heavily on the patient. The relationships that we create in life lead to the expectations from others on the roles that we play.

There are known chemical imbalances that can affect the ability to deal with stress. Keep in mind that our bodies tend to deal with stresses by the release of endogenous corticosteroids (natural steroids). The more the stress, the greater quantity of natural steroids that the adrenal glands produce. In times of reduced stress, it will down-regulate the formation and release of the natural corticosteroids. The true question to be answered is whether this chemical imbalance was the cause or the effect of the mind being overwhelmed with indecision and/or negativity.

Role of Perspective and Expectation

When we are discussing the body language of different viewpoints, we must give a proper role to that of context. Recognizing the normal steady state of a patient is necessary to establish whether someone is exhibiting more negativity than usual or rather just in their usual negative state. The same can be said of a person that appears happy but may indeed be normally even more demonstrably ecstatic. Where we consider the normal operating baseline is essential to the relative condition. This is a key point in being able to utilize body language awareness to both assess and to address deficiencies or imbalances in our relationships with patients. One of our main goals in bedside manner is to be able to positively affect healing in our patients by way of changing their perspective and teaching them to empower themselves through envisioning the fine details of a successful outcome. We all suffer from seemingly unfair judgments by others within and outside our normal social circles. Increasing our perspectives may help us see whether those judgments are valid or completely off base.

Many of our disappointments and successes in life revolve around the discrepancy between where we find ourselves and where we want to be. The expectation of an outcome colors our ideas of success and failure. The positive and negative sides both depend on where we are looking from. The power of these judgments to swing us from positive to negative or vice versa is key to our physical and emotional well-being. The entire empowering process involves envisioning a goal with all the details, looking for the opportunity in our everyday lives, and then finally taking the chance to embark on a different course. The exercise of committing to the ultimate goal can be a lifetime pursuit that we wish for ourselves and our loved ones. If we can manage the expectations of our patients to a realistic level and then stay on the positive perspective, we have done them a great service.

We need to allow that a mindset is a specific choice. If you decide prior to going on vacation that you will have a good time, the likelihood is that you will make the best of whatever situation in which you may find yourself. If your attention is distracted and you feel you'd rather be somewhere else, your vacation plans may be sabotaged. Your flexibility is a mindset that will greatly affect your idea of where you are and where you want to be. The expectation will frame a person's idea of success and thus adjust the judgment that comes along with success and failure.

Fishing for a "bite"

In the mentalist, psychic, and fortune-telling industry, there is a technique known as "cold reading." It employs a variety of methods to glean information about a person by careful observation as to their appearance, gender, education, religion, clothing, age, sexual orientation, and place of origin, among other factors. The mentalist or psychic then makes high-probability guesses to establish their credibility with the client. Due to a psychological quirk called confirmation bias (selectively hearing only what confirms our existing opinions), the clients often count the correct guesses and give little value to the incorrect ones. Rather than using these skills for profit, we can instead utilize these exceptional observation abilities to connect with the patients we serve.

As we initiate conversations, be mindful of the reactions that we elicit in those listening or actively speaking. Are they positive, negative, or undecided? The idea is to begin a conversation then look for the timely physical response in the form of body language. The body will react to something that does not yet rise to the level of eliciting a verbal response. When we hit upon a subject matter that finds a connection with a patient, their body language will show positive signs. This is a clear indicator to continue in this line of conversation. You may see a person "light up" with anticipation and eagerness to corroborate and elaborate upon their experience. Allowing them to add to the subject will strengthen the bond and allow you more information with which to further the conversation.

If we are clearly not hitting upon a subject of interest to the patient, the body language will remain negative without any energy placed into a response. It may feel much like talking to a log or a wall. Consider this as a sign to keep changing the channel until you hit upon an item or subject of interest. Do not consider it a failure if we only elicit negative body language, as you can still ascertain the issues that are not their main focus at this time. Keep in mind that the longer you take to find an item of interest, the connection that is initially present will begin to wane. There is certainly a time limit to any person's attention span.

More complicated is the undecided/unconvinced response, as it is somewhat negative in nature, but you may notice that the person maintains contact. This is the classic case of mixed signals. You may indeed have both positive and negative body language involved simultaneously. Neither one may be very emphatic. The effective response to this would be to shift slightly your subject to cover a different perspective yet making sure to not change the subject altogether. A shift in your angle of approach may give you more clues as to finding the necessary connection to proceed further.

In essence, this is an interplay of conversation that allows you to fine tune your connection, thus creating a friendly atmosphere for further communication. Should you hit upon a subject that instantly turns a person's body language negative, you will know that they feel strongly about the subject at hand. The idea is not to enter a vigorous debate situation (unless your goal is to provoke), but instead to find the connection with the patient that allows you access to help them heal. As healthcare practitioners, remember that we should not react to situations but instead respond after careful consideration of the different perspectives involved.

CHAPTER 3

Acquiring *the* Neutral Perspective *and the* Split Brain

When dealing strictly with the five senses of the human body, awareness allows us to take in and absorb raw information such as a person's appearance, the sound of their voice, or even the smell of a bacterial infection. With the increasing mass of information received, the need to interpret the data into patterns and an understandable rationale becomes apparent. This sorting of the details can be best viewed from what I call the *neutral perspective*. It is the place from which we can see the most perspectives of any situation. For example, every crime has a perpetrator, victim, unintended victims, as well as beneficiaries. If we are hearing the story from just the victim, it is from only one vantage point. Each and every patient also has a background that offers more perspectives. The more vantage points from which we look, the greater the advantage to sort out the stage at which illnesses or disorders begin.

The current standard of care states that we are to give "informed consent" to patients regarding their treatment options. This translates as providing choices for all the possible treatments for a given disease or disorder. While some cases can be limited to one or two options, others are significantly more complicated. Rather than only looking at the perspective of the patient, consider that of their spouse, child, or parent as well. Have they sought help for their problem before, or are they at the seventh attempt (not uncommon with smoking cessation) with different therapists and/or doctors? How has this affected their relationships with their loved ones, and has their role within their immediate family group changed because of their affliction? Essentially, we are tracking the course of their illness backwards from the time that we come into contact with the patient.

Outwardly, the neutral stance is perceived by patients to be nonjudgmental, which establishes a safe space for them to reveal their innermost thoughts behind their medical and personal histories. Physically and metaphorically creating this space is crucial to lay down mutually acceptable ground rules for engaging in the heavy work of healing. As it stands, healing can only be possible when a person is not actively engaged in surviving.

This neutral perspective has also been a central tenet of the more recent transcendental meditation movement, as well as traditional Buddhist teachings. In both, what I call the neutral perspective is a waypoint during the practice that opens up new ways to look at problems. It presents the perspectives of every participant in any event, showing the differing motivations, priorities, and expectations. Some may struggle to acquire this viewpoint, yet once achieved, the neutral perspective provides a vastly different view than what we are normally accustomed to.

As we begin to delve into the internals of the psyche, we need some background information to really appreciate the complexity of normal functioning processes. In order to understand how a patient may perceive our interactions, it helps to look at a rough model of the organization within the brain.

There is a common myth that our brains are divided into the left and right sides which serve different functions. This idea began in brain studies done by neuropsychologist Roger Wolcott Sperry, who worked with surgically treated epileptic patients who then subsequently lost other functions as well.[15] For his split-brain research, he was awarded the Nobel Prize in Physiology or Medicine in 1981. The central concept of his idea was that the left brain controls reasoning, logic, analytical, and critical thinking, while the right side controls music, emotions, intuition, and creative abilities. Although quite enduring, this idea is now considered a rather simplistic understanding of the extensive wiring of the brain. Anatomically, we can see from physiological studies that there are the left and right hemispheres and connections between the two. However, functions such as language are now known to exist on both hemispheres, and many tasks require that both sides work together intimately.

Figuratively speaking, I will retain the idea of the left brain, right brain—which together comprise the conscious mind—and the subconscious as a psychological differentiation, rather than a functional physiological one. There is a beauty in the simplicity of this three-node arrangement that is readily consumed and digestible. The fact that this delineation remains in our collective consciousness is testament to its inherent sway as an intuitive tool for teaching and learning.

The first node is the left brain, to which many individuals involved in technological careers are devoted. While an individual may have a preference and even a dominant side, we exist in a society that has abundant opportunities to train and develop the left brain functions. In the embrace of technology in our society, science and engineering courses of study are seen as precursors to professional careers, while art history and English literature graduates (on average) languish financially and struggle to find lucrative work. Many educational systems seem to place more resources on developing STEM (Science, Technology, Engineering, Math) graduates and somewhat secondarily, development of the creative mind.

The second node, the right brain, is no less important, and functions through the development of art through all its mediums, creation of music, and various creative uses of language abilities, i.e., poetry, literature, etc. It is a primary engine of what we consider to be pillars and hallmarks of culture. There seems to be an increasing emphasis in development of these skills after a period of general neglect. More opportunities are available to the development of the right brain now than during my formative periods in the 1970s through '90s.

There is a third integral component to the understanding of how we perceive the world. This is the integration of the subconscious brain, which learns long term skills and allows us to become increasingly efficient at a defined task. Much of the long-term memory is accessed through this portal, and it can be a storehouse for skills learned over a lifetime.

These three nodes of the brain: left brain, right brain, and the subconscious are operating concurrently at any given time depending on our perceived needs. We may simultaneously take in data from our five senses and then choose how to appreciate the analytical perspective (left brain), artistic qualities (right brain), and specific memory sequences required to repeat a given task (subconscious). As stated previously, most of us have a preference for how we choose to perceive any situation that is presented to us. Increased use of each area will exercise and train the associated node and thus strengthen the nerve connections within the physical brain that bolster the efficiency for that perspective.

These three components are all interconnected, and we are able to choose the point from which we begin perceiving the world. For example, if an automobile accident occurs in front of us during our morning commute to work, a left brain perception will concentrate on the facts of the crash, i.e., the severity of the crash, any injuries, how it affects the traffic, how much longer will it lengthen our commute. The right brain perception may look first at how it feels to be in an accident, how it sucks to be in heavy traffic, how it might feel to have injuries sustained in a crash. The subconscious may concentrate on a response to the accident such as preparing to stop to help if necessary, the rundown on steps for First Aid response, sequence of steps to CPR (cardiopulmonary resuscitation), or if the injuries are minor, switching out of the blocked lanes, moving out of the way of emergency vehicles, and calling into work to report a delay in arrival time. Further effects of the subconscious may be increased alertness with a heightened heart rate and a coursing of epinephrine through the circulatory system (the fight-or-flight response).

It is important to note that all the ways of perceiving the stimulus are valid, and we have a choice on how we take steps to act or react to any situation. Often we make the same choice repeatedly because it is familiar and comfortable. Thus we tend to favor one part of the brain over another in our interface with the world. With increasing usage of all the parts of the brain, the gaps between them will decrease, and eventually become a well-balanced functioning whole.

For patients seeking that connection with a doctor or healthcare practitioner who is sensitive to their needs, many intuitive qualities are already in play with regard to "comfort level" after meeting a new doctor. The gut feeling about the doctor may be the most effective subconscious-based tool to determine a good fit. Considering the volume of information that our subconscious minds take in on a regular basis, the gut feeling that it sends back to the conscious mind may be the most accurate way to gauge your overall comfort levels.

There is much variability in the capacity of a healthcare practitioner to listen. On top of that, people naturally have different personalities. Development of the social interpersonal skill set is uneven across the board. Trusting the intuition may feel alien to some, but humankind has lived many thousands of years without benefit of the information crush that we have today. The current emphasis on intellect should not be seen as a negative trait. Instead, healthcare practitioners must strengthen the ability to interpret messages from the subconscious (through feelings and other senses) to match the level of trust we have in our conscious brains (physical objective findings). This balancing of the left brain, right brain, and the subconscious are the basis upon which we can open up new ways of viewing old problems. When a doctor or healthcare worker can become responsive to patients on this level, patients can be confident that they have found someone to trust on a deeper level.

CHAPTER 4

Identity *and* Emotion

As medical professionals, we often concentrate on the treatment of the physical body (aside from mental health professionals), but often neglect the emotional side of healing. Rather than just a "bag of cells," our physical bodies are integrated into a complex network intertwined with our psyche and mind to combine into our idea of "self." In order to begin to shape our idea of the psyche and mind, it is helpful to think of each individual as a metaphorical container. This container has walls much like a drinking glass, and we choose the things that go inside as well as what remains on the outside. In other words, our self-image is shaped by the things or people for which we have an affinity as well as things or concepts that we admire.

For example, if I really enjoy baseball, I may choose to identify as a baseball player or baseball fan. As such, I place baseball inside my container and other competing sports on the outside. Whenever anyone brings up anything about the game of baseball, I can instantly relate to the information base and culture of baseball to engage in a spirited conversation. If someone happens to disparage the game of baseball, I would be inclined to defend the game, as I see it as part of my identity.

Another example may be the love of nature and outdoor environments. With multiple experiences that reinforce this very idea, we may choose to place this into our idea of self. The deeper the feeling of love for nature and the environment, the more it seeps into the container itself. Should another person engage in wanton pollution in the forest, or vandalism at a national park, we may begin to feel the need to defend against such an attack on something with which we identify strongly.

As we incorporate the ideas that we have included inside our container, items or concepts that we leave inside for a long time will begin to weave themselves into our actual decision-making process. We can see an increasing willingness to defend the things inside our container as if we were defending our physical selves from an attack. Should an actual attack occur against the things we hold dearest (concepts that are woven into our container), the attack becomes personal, and a physical as well as emotional response may result. The deeper the distress and insult to the current state of the container, the more dramatically the fight-or-flight response is triggered. Should the response tend toward fighting, the self-defense mechanisms kick in and the fur starts to fly. Should the insult be so invasive to the idea of self and any thought of turning back the attack seems unlikely, flight takes hold, and we retreat into our base emotions of fear and terror. The self will retreat into the memory of childhood and much of the reasoning and logic revert to a childhood state. Herein lies the difficulty in dealing with long standing phobias that drastically change the course of our lives. This retreat into a pre-developed state is one of the main reasons why fear elicits an irrational response.

We exist as a collection of choices that we have made over our immediate and long-term history. These choices are made throughout our lives to decide what our image of ourselves looks like. The things that we place inside our containers are items, people or concepts that become close to us. The walls of the container consist of the elements that make our decisions. Decisions that we continually renew then make their way into the very fabric of our container walls. You can even say that we are the container, along with everything we chose to be inside.

By contrast, all the things we leave outside our container will be casually discarded or forgotten over time. What we have decided to exclude from the container can also define our psyches.

During our physical and mental development, we often try on certain things for size within our containers. Initially, there is no permanence to the items we place inside our container unless we continually make the same choice. People may also decide to remove things from inside their container as they see fit. At the point of removal, they will no longer see it as part of themselves and likely will no longer see a need to defend it.

This very idea can be found in multiple spiritual traditions as there is a common acknowledgement of the inner self as a container (or house). Thus the development of the inner psyche is externalized into the physical world as the building of a house. One example is if a person strongly identifies with a naturopathic healing approach, they may think of modern pharmaceuticals as toxic mold in their house. Taking into consideration their sensibilities, we may steer them towards non-pharmacological and non-invasive means (fewer drugs and no surgery) and suggest lifestyle changes that achieve a similar goal. As practitioners, we need to keep this view of the inner self juxtaposed aside the physical body at the forefront of our minds as it plays a large role not just in how we communicate with our patients but also in the actual treatment plans we present.

Once we have established the complex construct of a person's identity, we then shift to what that identity is communicating through emotion. People often react to their emotions as a normal course of everyday life. Have you ever considered a piece of negative news received in the morning that affects your entire day? Perhaps you forget to complete an errand that puts you into a bad mood? This foul mood can wreak frustration, disappointment, or outright anger. None of us are immune to reacting to these emotions as if they were the original cause of the mood, which can then spiral into a self-fulfilling prophecy of creating a "bad day." Patients are not always aware that they display these emotions freely for others to pick up. Fortunately, healthcare practitioners are in a fine position to observe and assess these displays. When spotted, bringing this awareness to the patient may prevent a further downward spiral into something that already was a reaction itself.

More simply stated, frustration is an interpretation of unsatisfactory progress in an endeavor. Anger is a warning to others to prevent something undesirable from happening again. Fear is a caution of possible danger. Sadness is an expression of mourning. Happiness can be an expression of fulfillment of a goal or dream. Patient displays of external emotions may indeed be in conflict with their verbally stated declarations. The complexity of multiple simultaneous emotions may be present, or there may be a true internal conflict within. I cannot overstate the importance of this seemingly simple concept that we recognize emotions as a communication from the brain.

Many of us have experienced struggling with our emotions, and in inopportune moments have even changed the course of our lives when acting on them. The common rebuke, "Don't get emotional," is an oft-heard statement directed at someone about to cry. Traditionally, those of us who show their emotions and react to them are seen as weak and out of control. In our patriarchal society, the female gender has been maligned as the "weaker" sex for centuries with this very argument. For a number of my feminist-minded friends, this mischaracterization elicits outright anger. As another matter of observation, our past and current cultural consciousness of how a leader looks is remarkable for its stoicism, and lack of outward expression of any emotion. As such, emotions have been unfairly vilified due to a fundamental misunderstanding of its purpose and role in self-regulation of our individual psyches.

If we reframe emotions as a type of communication from our subconscious mind to our conscious minds, we will begin to see the complexity of our mental capacity for survival. Our subconscious mind operates and communicates by way of pictures, sounds, smells, tastes, and feelings.

It encompasses all five of our senses and may even account for many instances of the gut feeling. This gut feeling, and indeed most feelings, are interpretations of a core of information that is input into the subconscious. Due to the multitude of sensory inputs possible in any experience, our subconscious serves as a computer which takes in all the data then gives us a summary of what it thinks is happening overall. Should we have the bulk of the information point towards a dangerous situation, our subconscious mind will communicate this information with a feeling of danger and fear. It usually does not communicate through use of spoken language, as that is a learned human invention. When our conscious mind follows the message sent from the subconscious, we begin to see physiological changes associated with the active classical fight-or-flight response.

If your subconscious processes the information input and communicates a feeling of friendly familiarity, your conscious mind may seek to associate it with the feeling of being in your grandmother's old house or give you a feeling of déjà vu. Should your subconscious process a set of information that suggests grave injustice and unfairness, you may get the conscious mind message of depression followed by anger and revolt.

Karl Direske, a renowned teacher of healing based out of North Carolina, relates it best when he emphasizes the importance of "recognizing that these feelings are not the actual event but just a communication.[16]" When we can allow the communication and not kill the messenger, we may find that there is no immediate need to react to the message. We can take our time and contemplate the message prior to incorporating into our overall big-picture understanding of the situation. This allows us to reorganize our internal command structure to subordinate the information that we receive and then decide on an appropriate response rather than succumb to the snap reaction. When we can respond after careful consideration, we will effectively expand our choices for effectively dealing with a situation.

As a healthcare practitioner, you must keep your head level enough to avoid reacting to the emotions of patients. While we are all human and have our own daily struggles, we must take care to avoid treating a patient differently if we are experiencing our own difficulties. Should a patient be angry at a situation, it does no good to directly react to the anger. Compassion and empathy are certainly required to keep contact with the patient, but rather than react to their emotions, it is more effective to respond to the source of the anger. The most likely culprits may be impatience, misplaced expectations, or loss of control.

Many people are accustomed to a certain reaction in others when they show anger, sadness, frustration, or happiness. It is not uncommon for a supervisor or other upper management to use their emotional outbursts to "motivate" their workers. Remember that as healers, we stand independent from the social or occupational standing of our patients. We need only to respond to the underlying communication that brought forth the emotion.

CHAPTER 5

How Our Brains Learn

A s we begin to move inwards from verbal communication to body language to the psyche, recognize that there are corresponding neurological actions that dictate the physiological response that we witness. In delving deeper into the neurological process, we can see that there are evolutionary advantageous reasons to the existing mechanisms. This chapter lays the groundwork for later discussion on how certain common disorders can hijack the normal mechanisms and distort the downstream effects. Understanding these processes allows us to trace backwards from how a patient presents to us and eventually ferret out how they developed that way.

In attempting to unravel the complex patterns of short-term and long-term learning that manifest themselves as connections within the physical brain, we will need to grasp the basic mechanisms involved. Although much remains to be discovered, we have come to understand some basic operations. Experiences are recorded within our brains as two main types of memory: explicit and implicit. Explicit memory retains the conscious information such as names, dates, people, places, and objects. We can further categorize the explicit (sometimes called declarative) memory into personal, episodic memory and factual, semantic memory. Details about a movie date or a promise made to your daughter would be kept in the episodic memory, while the date and time of a football game or concert would be a semantic memory. This engages the hippocampus and medial temporal lobe areas in the brain. Implicit memory includes recollections of things and procedures that are not in the conscious realm, such as walking or riding a bicycle. Typically, the cerebellum and the striatum are active when performing these tasks.

Our brains take in sensory input en masse into the explicit short-term memory, called *working memory*, which initially lasts from 20 to 30 seconds.[17] Within this duration, your brain decides whether the information is important enough to retain over a longer period. The actionable elements are then consolidated into the conscious long-term memory, which occurs over several hours. The remainder of the collected information that does not achieve conscious long-term status then resides in the subconscious level. Sleep has been shown to both enhance the memories that the brain wants to keep and assist in forgetting the ones that are deemed impertinent.[18] Physically, the long-term memory is then stored by way of new synaptic connections into the neocortex, the wrinkly outer surface of the brain.

Note that there are two separate processes ongoing at this sorting stage. One is the consolidation of short to long-term memory, which happens mostly in the hippocampus. In the other pathway, which neurologists refer to as salience, the information most relevant to survival is brought to attention. It is a primitive survival mechanism that channels directly to the amygdala, two almond-shaped areas of gray matter at the base of both cerebral hemispheres, which ingrains each memory with emotional significance. A whole branch of psychology called evolutionary psychology is devoted to how these survival mechanisms still manifest themselves in our modern behavior despite no longer having to spend every moment devoted to survival.[19] As our modern physical surroundings having undergone tremendous change compared with the hunter-gatherer stage of human development, particular behaviors such as boasting, rage, lying, vanity, promiscuity, and many others are still encoded into our DNA.

These behaviors that once improved early human fitness for survival and gene propagation account for a significant portion of our social dysfunctions today.

From a psychological standpoint, most long-term memory is stored in the subconscious mind, along with the automatic responses to specific situations that are trained. We spend most of our time in the conscious state that allows the left brain and right brain to interact via our intelligence and emotion. Again, there needs to be a distinction made between the psychological terms of left brain, right brain, and subconscious brain versus the neurological regions represented by the anatomical structures— frontal lobe, prefrontal cortex, amygdala, medial temporal lobe, etc. As there continues to be ongoing investigations that show the extreme complexity of how the brain is physically wired, our discussion mainly centers around the psychological organization instead. In other words, the subconscious brain to which we refer may actually be in several regions of the anatomical brain.

As such, it is useful to be familiar with some of the sophisticated tools with which much research continues. Brain research scientists have utilized modern imaging tools such as PET scans (positron emission tomography) to discover the pathways that information is processed. Considering that all cells, including those in the brain, are fed by glucose, usage of radioactive-tagged glucose will be revealed on the PET scans. As the brain is engaged specific activities, we can then see which parts of the brain are working as they will utilize more fuel in the form of glucose. Another tool, the fMRI (functional magnetic resonance imaging) is used to detect the changes in blood flow through the small capillaries in the brain under different conditions. Similarly, any incremental increase in blood flow during an activity will show that a specific part of the brain is actively engaged.

In general, vast amounts of information are gathered by the subconscious mind, then the most relevant and important points are passed onto the parts of the left and right brain for decision-making. It appears that there are certain topics that are automatically passed through as salient. These include what we affectionately call the three Fs: Feeding, Fighting (fight-or-flight), and F*cking. Keep a mental note as this will become important in our discussion of coping and addictions.

Through constant sensory input in our infancy and childhood, we develop patterns that are interpreted as beneficial or damaging. Some events, however, are not as impactful and are then stored away in the general memory of our subconscious. The subconscious serves as a main hard drive that stores all our sensory inputs while the conscious mind is activated for immediate survival and other active cognition. As we begin to encounter the same or similar situations, our recognition of the circumstance begins to process the proper response that will keep us alive. Over the course of repetition, the situation and its proper response are shifted from the active conscious mind into the more organized part of the hard drive, which is the area for subconscious learning. This subconscious learning eventually allows us to draw the proper response to a familiar situation with increasing speed. The traumas and phobias that are repeatedly triggered will have a priming effect much like that of a sprinter who is well trained for a 100-meter dash. The pathways that are utilized often will be reactivated with greater speed and efficiency than an unprimed pathway.

Despite some controversy, one of the popular ideas from Malcolm Gladwell's book *Outliers*[20] considers the idea that repetition for 10,000 hours will result in the optimum speed of response to any learned activity. Of course, the huge variability of talent and innate predispositions to a specific activity will often determine the speed of learning. In general, there is little argument that practice will improve any task relative to a complete beginner.

There is also a type of learning called conditioning. The mind draws associations between things that occur repeatedly and predictably at the same time. The classic example of this conditioning is the example of Pavlov's dog. In his experiments with canines, Ivan Pavlov rang a bell each time he fed the dogs in his study. He carefully measured the amount of saliva produced at baseline, then again at feeding time. With repetition, he found that just the act of ringing the bell elicited salivation in the dogs.

Over the course of the years extending through childhood and adolescence, our learned responses start to emerge as larger patterns. Every family with children will have witnessed the vagaries of certain favorite foods (e.g. hamburgers and pizza) as well as things that are avoided like the plague (broccoli and brussels sprouts, anyone?). We will actively need to use the conscious mind to look back into our subconscious to make sense of these patterns. Patterns that are strongly reinforced through repeated learning cycles become incorporated as a belief within the subconscious mind. Once beliefs are passed back to the conscious mind, we tend to shape and color our sensory inputs with what we have come to believe.

We have all had instances of friends and relatives who selectively hear what they want to hear. The term *confirmation bias* describes exactly this tendency of even highly intelligent individuals to favor and interpret information that already confirms their beliefs.[21] Items that do not match their beliefs are conveniently deprioritized and underreported to the conscious mind. We then start to see opinion-based "truths" treated as facts.

It takes an extremely balanced individual to go back to the conscious mind and allow new sensory inputs to continue to shape their subconscious rather than the other way around. Facts are learned truths that can be proven with scientific evidence, and the proof needs to be indefinitely repeatable as necessary for edification of the conscious mind. However, belief does not need to rise to the level of "fact" in order for it to be considered a "truth" by a person. "Truths" may indeed only be opinions from the viewpoint of one or more person's experience.[22]

From the neurological perspective, the dopamine pathway comes into the discussion when we look at its role as the reward center. Recall its involvement in the evolution of dog eyes muscles in Chapter 2. Currently, dopamine is one out of over one hundred neurotransmitters identified in the brain so far, most of which have not been extensively studied. As noted previously, there are basic functions, including the three Fs, that activate our reward systems. In fact, any number of activities that can be considered enjoyable are activating this pathway. Dopamine is released by neurons as part of an excitatory pathway. Between each neuron there is a space called the synapse. An electrical signal passing from one nerve cell to the next stimulates the nerve ending to release dopamine across the synapse. The next neuron which contains dopamine receptors is activated when the released dopamine reaches and binds to these receptors. As this excitatory signal conducts along multiple neurons, it ultimately reaches an area in the brain called the *nucleus accumbens*, which results in a torrent of excitatory pleasure. There are other areas of the brain associated with this reward response, including but not limited to the ventral tegmental area, striatum, amygdala, insula, and subgenual anterior cingulate cortex. For our purposes, the distinction of each brain region is not critical, but it is important to note that individual functions may exist in multiple parts of the brain. The neurons involved in these reward pathways are stimulated by a trigger, which varies based on what we perceive as satisfying the "salient" needs, as well as things that reaffirm the nature of our individual containers.

It is important to note that there is an opposite sedative pathway right alongside the dopamine pathway. In other neurons, another neurotransmitter, γ-aminobutyric acid (GABA), provides the opposite effect to dopamine.[23] Many of the popular anesthetic medications (propofol, etomidate, methohexital, thiopental, isoflurane, sevoflurane, and desflurane) activate this pathway for anesthesia and sedation. There is evidence that this pathway can act independently or as a method of attenuation of the excitatory dopamine pathway. In other words, it can work alone or for the purpose of balancing dopamine.

These excitatory and inhibitory pathways are important due to their prominence in shaping our personalities as well as learning experiences. We can start to draw together the psychological observations and relate them to the dopamine reward pathway. For example, a person learning to play a musical instrument is attracted to the sound of the music. Listening to the music activates the reward pathway and floods the nucleus accumbens with dopamine, eliciting a rush of pleasure. Cognitively, the association of music and pleasure is established. Practicing with the instrument then allows the learner to hear bits and pieces of the sound emanating from their mental map of the musical piece on which they are working. Further identification with musicians and the experience of playing their chosen instrument strengthens their identity as a musician. The reward pathway at various levels is stimulated at each step of their progress as a musician.

What is remarkable, if only for its simplicity, is the idea that we can choose our own mental image of ourselves. This becomes the basis upon which our reward system is applied. Somewhere along the path of the maturing mind of a child, a certain threshold of basic learning is passed when our inner judge begins to develop. The idea of self and the ego come into play, and we begin to decide what is internal and what remains external. This process helps us sort a massive amount of sensory information that comes through our five senses.

When we examine the basic learning process of the human mind, we can also observe how people receive "good" versus "bad" new information. What is the significant factor when judging whether something is deemed good or bad? It appears that humans judge new sensory input to be good when it matches their perception of how things should be, reminds them of a previous positive experience, and/or reinforces what they already believe, regardless of whether it is a hard fact or an opinion-based truth. As the good perception feeds the ego, we see activation of the dopamine reward pathway. Psychologists refer to this need for regular feeding of the ego as the "hedonic treadmill." We see the dopamine feedback cycle employed by multiple social media companies in controlling what news articles appear on our daily feed.[24]

Conversely, "bad" news tends to be incongruent with our existing belief of how things should be, based on our previous learning. Clearly, input that directly conflicts with our pre-programmed truth will be judged as incompatible and unacceptable. This judgment either leads us to reject the news as untrue (denial) or will cause us to reexamine our truths. Thus, as health practitioners, we have an inherent difficulty when delivering bad news that patients do not want to hear. In these instances, the dopamine reward system is suppressed, and the areas of memory associated with previous instances of bad news is stimulated and replayed.[25]

During psychological development, the idea of self and the container that separates the external from the internal is established. We become the container and decide what elements to identify with as self and what elements don't fit within this idea of self. This is essential to the growth and healthy development of every human being. Children have a visceral need to try out different combinations of things to include on the inside and specifically what to exclude, eventually coming to a fairly steady state of who they want to be at a particular point in time.

With the continuing development of the idea of self and ego, we see the simultaneous emergence of the inner judge which is tasked with deciding what fits and what is out of place. Once the ego is somewhat stable and the judge is confident enough in its ability to choose comfortably, we find the emergence of free will. This free will represents choice and exists in a nascent stage prior to the awareness of self, ego-realization, and the establishment of the judge. Once we have the idea of self, then comes the ability to shape our future learning through the choice of free will.

Through this developmental stage, any disruption or trauma is usually remembered as a major event, as there are not many other events with which to compare. Often, the monumental aspect of this event is combined with an external judgment from the parents and family surrounding the child. As the parents or family are directly in contact with the child, their response to the trauma becomes the sensory input for the child. This external judgment, being most likely negative in nature, takes on a large role, since the internal judge of the child is not yet independent and confident nor fully developed. The nascent mind asks the questions of "what happened?" and "why?" and "did I do something wrong?" and "is it my fault?" This in turn nurtures the idea that something is wrong, and the negativity that results is repeated in the mind of the child.

These questions either persist without an answer or are given an answer that is cobbled together to make sense to a child's immature mind. Whatever the reason, it is repeated in the mind of the child from their perspective. The repetition of this negative event unknowingly becomes a learned response, just as surely as a baseball player throws a baseball repeatedly to learn a new pitch. Inadvertently, the child becomes an expert at this negative event or trauma. However, they experienced it without the benefit of a mature resolution. In this manner, childhood traumas that occur during this developmental period have a way of persisting in the lives of those involved.

We may yet find that many adult mental health issues have their origins in these negative experiences as children. Being experts at the trauma and having relived it multiple times in their mind, children amplify the downstream reactions to any similar event in the future. Phobias, fixations, addictions, and judgments all have their roots in these types of situations early on in life. In fact, these early traumas all seem to be more impactful than later traumas of similar types. It is in the response to the trauma that we find differences between a mind arrested in development versus a mature adaptable mind that can overcome the issue and eventually heal. We will need to address the proper and complete healing of these early life events to truly understand some deep-seated issues.

Some of these experiences that have been explained with the rationale from a child's perspective will explain why many of us have habits and idiosyncrasies that do not have a basis in logic. Without resolution of these issues, our minds find a workaround, and these lead to the formation of phobias, addictions, and other non-useful psychological dysfunctions that change the course of our lives.

When we examine the nature of these dysfunctions more carefully, they seem to follow a distinctive pattern. For the most part, most of them are pre-programmed solutions to a particular situation. It is likely that these solutions once worked for the situation at the time of initial occurrence. However, the solution that previously worked may no longer be the appropriate response. Therefore, application of the previous program to a current situation that slightly resembles the similar original situation is no longer working.

For example, let us consider a childhood episode with a spider bite. The poison in the spider venom may have caused significant pain, suffering, and a very unpleasant trip to the local emergency room. The mind subsequently inserts a healthy fear of spiders, and the child repeats this fear over and over in their mind until the fear attains manic proportions. This phobia to even non-poisonous spiders may even become an impedance to a normal life. Provided there is no new sensory input to replace or add to that of the initial poisonous spider bite, it is likely this phobia will exist for many years or even decades. What was once a useful psychological program for self-preservation is amplified through repetition, imagination, and time. As an adult, this may even lead the individual to avoid natural settings or develop an unhealthy habit of cleaning excessively.

Over the course of our lives, we will have made millions of conscious choices on top of the multiple billions made by our subconscious mind that are based on our deepest-set ideas of truths. When we look at the value of learned experience over a lifetime and consider the commutations and permutations of choices we make, we as individuals are indeed unique in every way.

CHAPTER 6

A Walk Down Memory Lane

When we discuss medical history with patients, they usually do not express their personal history in an impartial manner. It may be full of opinions and biases as well as significant blame on people or things out of their control. There is an appropriate need to filter out some of the personal angles in order to ascertain what really happened to them. There is a great deal to be had in understanding the process by which memory forms within our brains.

Other than the current moment, every other happening and event in our lives involves our memory. While the future requires an imagination and visualization, everything that makes up our personal and collective history is stored in the dendritic connections of our brain. From the moment we have consciousness, our memory is the key pathway by which we learn how to survive and interact with the world around us. Even while still in the uterus, human fetuses have the capacity to learn rhythms and sounds and recognize the mother's voice.[26] Given the current popularity of DNA databases that link genealogies, there is ample interest in where we came from, which appears to give context to who we are now. Our memory shapes our idea of ourselves and often give meaning to our lives. However, research shows that we also shape our memories to fit our idea of who we are.

From our earliest moments in infancy, there is recognition of the breast or bottle of milk that satisfies hunger, the face of your mother that signifies comfort and protection, the shape and sounds of other children that hint of playtime and laughter. Clearly, memory exists and is working in the developing brain of an infant and child. It is thus particularly interesting that at the age of 3 years, the active autobiographical memory of the infant is forgotten only to give way to the earliest childhood memories. In the scientific literature, this significant loss of memory is widely known as *infantile amnesia*.[27] If one episode was not enough, this amnestic phenomenon occurs again at about the age of 7 years and has been coined *childhood amnesia*. While the reason for these episodes of mass memory loss is not well known, we do know that they coincide with periods of development of rapid increases in overall memory capacity. It is also suspected that this is related to a failure in the consolidation step of memory storage.[28] The peculiar aspect is that this memory loss is concentrated on the autobiographical episodic memory and not necessarily the semantic memory.[29] In other words, the child may remember how to play with a toy but have no conscious information about who gave them the toy or the occasion on which they received it. It seems that the more rapidly the brain grows to increase capacity, it is also shedding old memories even faster.

When we consider all that is lost, we are still left with the remnants of the retained memory. There is ample evidence that early life memories and experiences have significant effects on predispositions to later developmental and psychiatric disorders.[30] There are also countless cases of lifelong phobias that generated from childhood situations, much like the instance of the spider bite.

One major clue as to what memories are deemed worthy of being retained from short-term to long-term was discussed by Patricia Bauer in her 2014 study on childhood amnesia.[31] Parents were instructed to ask their children to recall an event that occurred recently. They were given a choice to either acknowledge them by restating what the child said or to inquire more about the event. When children were asked by their parents to elaborate on their narratives and were asked to "tell me more" about the event, the children consistently recalled more details about the event. The act of repeating their impressions and feelings of the event apparently gave them more data points to help associate with the experience. This association with the smells, sounds, and feelings with the event created a diverse combination of specific details with connections to multiple sensory organs. The greater the number of sensory inputs, the greater the recall, especially with smell.[32]

Another significant finding is the discovery that the mind can incorporate a false memory as a data point in its own internal narrative. There appears to be a psychological need to fill in the blanks from times in our lives when our memory is insufficient. This urge exposes this frailty in human memory by taking snippets of images and photographs and then stitching them with statements from other people about their experience to create a fictionalized memory imbued with details, depth of feeling, and even humor.[33] It is due to this phenomenon that eyewitnesses cannot always be relied upon in a court of law.[34]

In our context of healing, the recognition of amplification and omission errors in memory, as well as recollection of events especially in cases of anxiety, stress, or phobias, allows us to strike a position of accepting differing perceived realities as experienced by the patient versus that of the healthcare practitioner. We do not necessarily need to assert our observations as the only truth when we can simply state, "I see how you can remember it that way."

CHAPTER 7

Practical Application *of* Heightened Awareness

Returning to Ella's statement of wanting to "smile again," we discovered that she suffers not only from the physical condition of poor dental health but also a culmination of guilt, shame, and depression, leading to breakdowns in her interpersonal relationships. At the time, she reported smoking one pack of cigarettes per day for thirty years (self-reporting usually underestimates by quite a bit). Unfortunately, this is an all-too-common occurrence in our daily practice. We witness the ongoing "works in progress" that present as a jumble of psychological issues that further complicate one or more physical illnesses. At this point, it would be natural to feel a hesitance to delve further into this patient relationship as the variables beyond our control can be quite staggering. However, we would be remiss in assuming that Ella's difficulties are beyond help.

As we continue to look for openings in our dialogue and uncover clues to the unspoken meaning of her words, we seem to hit a vein of deep feeling. In response to a question about when the last time she felt confident with her smile, she pauses poignantly and nostalgically declares, "I remember having a beautiful smile that all my teenage friends envied!" Through careful conversation and the expression of the awareness skills that we have discussed, we trace Ella's self-esteem issues to her late teenage years with the traumatic loss of her mother. It became apparent that she still harbored repressed emotions and inwardly mourned from that pivotal time in her life despite the many decades that have passed.

Observing her general appearance, her clothing is conservative, clean, and well pressed, which indicates a desire to present well and shows self-respect. There appears to be an underlying sadness to her overall demeanor, telegraphing her complex story. Reading her body language, she has downcast eyes, frequently avoiding contact, with occasional twitching, possibly hiding significant discomfort and embarrassment. However, her open shoulder and hip stance indicates that she is willing to engage more to reveal her complicated history. Thus a little deeper probing is warranted. Avoiding placing any judgment on her current condition, she carefully relates her life experiences with emotions as if it had happened yesterday. She explains that her depression followed her mother's untimely death, and she expresses a feeling of overwhelming responsibility for caring for her widowed father. This in turn led her to start smoking as a stress reliever. The smoking serves as the coping mechanism that allows her to relieve some stress yet has multiple negative effects on her dental and overall health.

Maintaining the safe space, we offer gentle cues of affirmation, encouraging her to continue. Our expressions of compassion as well as our ability to relate resonate with Ella. In validating her feelings, as well as reflecting back to her our observations on her tone, body language, and expressions, she feels a safe connection that facilitates further sharing of her story. It is apparent that she regards her mother's death as a turning point in her life when she began to feel the weight of the world. At the time, her dental health was a distant priority in the face of survival. She had always had a beautifully genuine smile, and it never occurred to her that her perceived strength could evolve into a shame. Her Christian faith sustains her, yet she feels that she has fared poorly as a wife. Over the course of several decades and two failed marriages, her self-esteem took a battering and her self-care waned.

Ella's dental problems were an end-stage manifestation of poor home care or even neglect stemming from many factors. Her dental dysfunctions were likely connected to her overall self-esteem which in turn adversely affected her hygiene habits and food choices. As a result of uninformed food choices, she suffered from poor diabetes control, cholesterol imbalance, and unwanted weight gain.

Ensnared in an endless struggle, she learned in bits and pieces what she could about health and medicine over the years. Without having the scientific background nor emotional support to guide her on a daily basis, she lacked the information and support structure to gauge the location of her balance points. Fortunately, amidst her struggle, she managed to successfully raise two daughters, who were now financing her medical treatment.

When considering the challenges Ella faced, we can best further her progress by defining the manner in which we can help, thereby limiting the scope of work necessary. At the same time, recognize that recovery in one aspect may affect another variable that could well be out of our personal expertise. This framing of the specific problem places the healthcare practitioner into the position of a guide to health, rather than the sole vehicle to healing. We can impress the idea that success within our limited scope serves as one brick on the road to a greater recovery. Providing this type of structure allows the patient to see healing as a process with which we are helping them, yet requiring their personal investment and judgment. Another criterion will be matching the tone and energy levels of the patient. The urgency for resolution of their problem must be gauged in order to determine the extent of their commitment. At what stage of the healing process are they currently engaged? Have they suffered greatly from the effects of their illness and are at the end of their patience, or are they just at the beginning of gathering information? How aggressive or conservative are they in their approach? What is their expected pace of treatment? These are some of the important questions that will determine your approach.

As for the energy levels, how proactive do they expect you to be? Even if you cannot immediately solve the problem, your pace of troubleshooting should be in tune with the patient's expectations. Starting with a neutral stance, adjust your speed of progression to match their pace. While working through your diagnosis and treatment flow chart, assess their deficiencies, whether it be knowledge, money, time, and/or desire. Feed the deficiency by systematically addressing their main areas of concern. This does not mean that you need to perfectly match the patient's expectations. It will suffice to be complementary to their tone and energy levels. For example, if they are lacking in motivation, you can complement them by creating a structure and plan for them to make progress. If they are reckless in their pursuit of an answer, you can provide stability in their options, yet still respect their time frame.

Conventional therapy, at this point, dictates the formulation of a treatment plan. Provided we consider all the aspects that are most important to the patient, how do we achieve a plan that allows the patient to fully buy into the process? Aside from the nuts and bolts of the treatment plan, a patient's belief in your ability to help them makes a tremendous effect on our eventual success rates.

As we are only starting to put together the big picture for the pathways involved in human behavior, recognize that there are many neurotransmitters working alone and in concert to affect our behavior. What is clear is that there are many factors involved in our habits and compulsions. At the center of all this neurology and biochemistry, is still our ability to choose and the reasons we have for doing so. Seeing through the main motivations and removing the layers of guilt, shame, and judgment will allow us to virtually walk into the working minds of our patients. If we choose to share our observations with them, we may begin to condition our patients to feel better after every visit.

PART 2

Cultivating Belief

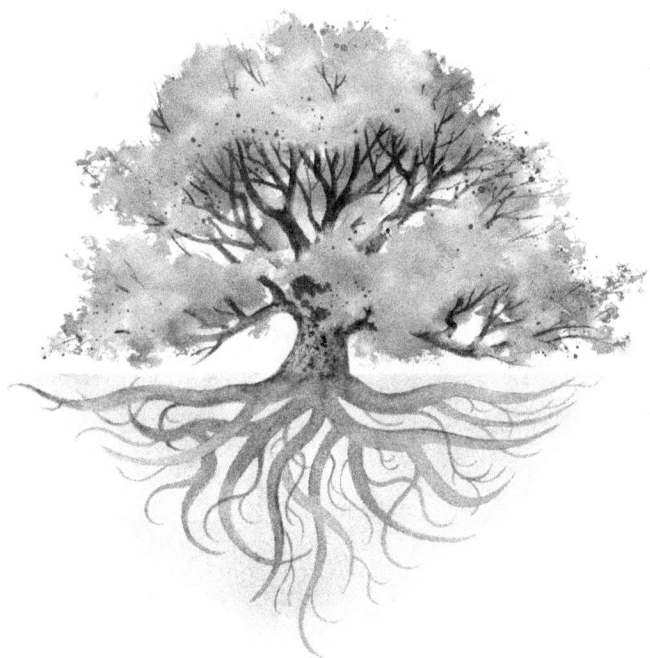

In studying the power of belief, we need look no further than the great spiritual traditions of the world. Literature and film are abounding with stories of devout believers achieving seemingly impossible tasks. Every known major spiritual tradition deals in the teaching of some specialized wisdom that is not in wide discourse. The knowledge is revealed slowly over time, as understanding of the esoteric concepts require earnest learning. After significant effort at mental digestion, these uncommon insights then develop into wisdom that provides an explanation to the fundamental existential questions of life. The common thread between these traditions is this special insight that speaks to the universal human condition.

There is even debate that this need for belief may be coded in our genetics.[35] While it is now considered quite simplistic to attribute the human need for belief into one single gene, we are still left wondering whether our genes in concert affect or even enable our spirituality. There exists an ongoing philosophical debate regarding whether we as humans have a greater spiritual and scientific need for religion or whether religion itself needs us as followers more. As these debates will naturally elicit strong reactions, we can nevertheless be assured that there will continue to be many gray areas which will challenge our belief systems. However, we can contend that the power of spirituality lies in the insight and foresight of the teachings. Consider the possibility that we can tap into and engage the combination of genes and conscious choice which follow the evolution from initial confidence to trust, from trust to belief, then again from casual belief to solid conviction.

Deep in the indigenous villages of the Amazon, shamanic healers still challenge the belief systems of all manner of afflicted souls. Of particular note are the shamans dealing with the hallucinogenic plant mixture called ayahuasca. Concocted mainly with the *Banisteriopsis caapi* vine and the leaves of *Psychotria viridis*, the tea mixture is boiled and concentrated to amplify the psychotropic effects.[36] Alone, each plant has a mild effect, lasting approximately 10–30 minutes.[37] Yet combined, there is a synergy, magnifying the psychoactive effects of each (peaking between 90–120 minutes) and extending the duration to about 4 hours.[38]

Western seekers of these shamans are often people who have been failed by modern medicine and have been forced to expand their horizons on the complexity of their illnesses. Upon arriving to the healer of their choosing, patients are subject to examination on the nature of their problems and their backgrounds.[39] A prescribed period of cleansing must be followed to isolate their illness, which may include extended fasting, forest bathing, herbal preparations, and purging. Along the way, a diagnosis is developed after immersing the patient in a world where the plants themselves communicate to both the healer and the patient. In an overnight ceremony, ayahuasca is ingested under the watchful eye of the shaman.

With the help of the hallucinogenic herbal tea, a hyper-conscious (some may call it semi-conscious) state of mind is achieved. However, the side effects cannot be underestimated, as they can include vomiting, diarrhea, hallucinations, out-of-body experiences, fear, paranoia, and euphoria. Many that have gone through the healing ceremony have reported the transcendence of time and space, meeting of sentient beings, a sense of oneness, traveling in a tunnel toward a light, and even a life review (usually associated with near-death experiences.)[40] Considering that the effects vary between each ingestion and can be different for each individual, the guiding force and experience of the shaman will often determine a patient's success or failure. The ceremony's songs and prayers all express the specifics of the healing as prescribed by the plant communication.

Whereas the diagnosis, prescription, and follow-up are familiar steps of the healing process, the ayahuasca ceremony is remarkable for its head-first dive into an elaborate belief system and world view that requires a severe departure for most Western patients. The major leap necessary to enter this world is the indigenous belief that the plants themselves have a consciousness and are actively directing the healing of the patient. The source of the heightened awareness is actually the spirit of the plants. In a sense, the shaman is serving as the guide and translator for the plant spirits. The emotional, cognitive, and physical effects appear to be beneficial for many of the illnesses where Western medicine still lags, such as addiction, depression, anxiety, and other psychiatric imbalances.[41] If the indigenous belief system is not adopted, the desired healing effects are not likely to be fruitful. There is no question that the intense period of internal examination has a healing effect in these cases. However, the many patients that have seen success from ayahuasca shamans universally have an altered and widened world view.

Belief is still as much a part of traditional healing as it is in the modern day, yet we consistently fail to engage our patients in this manner in contemporary medical and dental settings. As practitioners of evidence-based, science-rooted Western medicine, we may be loath to admit that belief plays a significant role in the health outcomes of our patients. But like it or not, it very much plays a meaningful role in healing, and to help our patients to the best of our abilities we must fully engage with their belief systems.

If we, as modern-day healers, can harness our observation and awareness skills to the point of acuity, we can then share our unique insight into the nature of our patients' illnesses. In other words, we can strengthen a causal connection to become a belief when we are able to show the details of what we see in a person's everyday presentation. Our perceptiveness becomes the tool by which we can convince a person of our ability to help them. When we identify and address the idiosyncrasies and behavioral patterns that are associated with each patient, we can then process the manner in which they can best receive the information.

I recall a conversation that I had with a friend who worked for a global positioning system (GPS) company at the time. He was involved in beta testing of portable automobile GPS units and had set the test unit to a female voice that resembled that of his long-time spouse. According to him, he kept missing the driving instructions. Apparently, he automatically tuned out what sounded like her voice. Once he discovered this quite unintentional conditioning of his subconscious mind, he was able to remedy the situation. In his case, my friend had a preconditioned existing preference for a voice that was different from his wife's. Although their relationship was quite outwardly loving, he regularly complained about his wife nagging him. Regardless of whether we feel a need to judge his relationship, his conditioning represents the same biases that our patients will exhibit when seeking medical help. This will be a key part of the puzzle for us to figure out how we can best communicate in a way that will elicit the desired moment of revelation.

We are interpreting vast amounts of data that we have collected into a friendly succinct summary to be presented in the most palatable manner. With the additional histories of the patients, we can project over time and even develop a foresight into the likely individual futures of our patients. When we present our awareness-enhanced perspectives (including observations and previous experiences), our goal is to win over the trust of a patient, eventually evoking a belief in both our ability to cure their condition as well as their own ability to heal. In these days of easy access to various questionable sources on the Internet, scientific evidence alone may not be adequate to engage a person's belief systems. The whole package gleaned from medical training, acute awareness, and empathetic communication may be necessary to bridge the gap.

If we achieve this level of belief, there is no question that patients are significantly more compliant with aftercare instructions and will have a more positive attitude towards pain and the entire healing process.[42] They will also recognize your role in working for their benefit, thus minimizing instances of them working against your recommendations either consciously or subconsciously.

When we are developing a treatment plan for a patient, we should aim for a strong connection that not only addresses the chief complaint but also includes details and what may seem minor but are essential pivotal factors in the process. We must communicate the extent of our detailed observations and juxtapose them with our known models of health. In thoroughly explaining the existing dysfunction, and directly comparing it with the "normal" state, we draw a direct line that marks the path to resolution of the illness. This imparting of information, the product of careful observation, serves not only as education for the patient, but ties into the cultivation of their belief system. We are providing not only the same widely available information found on the Internet but essentially showing them the much greater value for visiting a highly trained professional in person. This bond borne from trust is then allowed to grow into belief with repeated successes.

Often the pervasive problem of non-compliant patients is simply blamed on unruly behavior. This common lamentation on patients not following directions still echoes loudly in schools, hospitals, and residencies worldwide. What is actually happening is much more likely an inadequate engagement of the patient's belief systems. When a patient arrives at the realization that you are an essential part of a team devoted to their well-being, their confidence in you becomes a foundational conviction.

CHAPTER 8

Establishing Contact *and* Connection

I n the contemporary context, we no longer regularly rely on mysticism as a viable method to engage a person's belief system. However, the human brain still relies on instincts that are vestiges of an evolutionary process that remains despite not being adapted to our modern surroundings. Journalist, author, and professor Robert Wright likes to refer to the example of road rage. On the evolutionary context, rage (a level of anger that exceeds the appropriate circumstance) was once useful in the tribal community because it showed to others that you were not one to be wronged. In a sense, a person's rage was a communication to others that there are negative consequences to offending you. That trait of explosive anger that prevents future offenses is then passed onto future generations.

In the modern day, we can commonly see this rage in the form of road rage, especially when stuck in rush hour traffic. Intellectually, we know that we are not statistically likely to see the same people driving in cars next to us, yet the anger and the compulsion to rage at the person who just cut in front of you remains.

There is often a snap decision that is made upon meeting a new person often referred to as the first impression. As many of us know from experience, the initial thoughts about an individual often shape how we feel about them regardless of whether our impressions turn out to be true. We tend to favor those with whom we have similarities. Evolutionary psychologists call this behavior 'tribalism,' which includes a fairly rapid decision on whether a new person that you meet can be trusted or should be resisted. This behavior is coded into our genetics for the purpose of survival. Indeed, it has prominently shaped our ideas of history, civilization, and politics from the beginnings of recorded consciousness.[43]

The difficulty for healthcare workers (and pubescent teens, for that matter) lies in the stubbornness of initial impressions. It raises the stakes of every initial interaction with patients and makes the consequences of negative outcomes linger. As such, making contact with a patient in a controlled manner that minimizes negative consequences has much appeal.

At the initial presentation of any health issue, we are often lacking in time to get acquainted. Many patients will deal with any discomfort, pain, and inconvenience until the point where they feel it is persisting and worsening. As such, our entrance into the history of the patient's medical problem will need to fill in the blank spaces particularly in establishing any known signs and symptoms.

Where the patient stands from a degree of exasperation will often determine their initial willingness to comply with your recommendations. In other more chronic situations, patients will have already developed a coping mechanism that allows them to avoid some of the discomfort and pain, but not eliminate it altogether. Should you have a very compliant patient, your job of doctoring and healing becomes fairly straightforward. However, some patients have a strong sense of where they want their treatment to lead. If they have a solid idea of the actual cause and diagnosis, you are once again in a fortunate position. The suggested treatment may well be familiar to both patient and healthcare practitioner. In the instance where the patient has a misguided idea of the cause, we may need to wrestle with how deeply ingrained their initial ideas color their understanding. Indeed, there may be a challenge to your status as someone who can help them. You may have a patient who only wants you to perform a procedure that they have already determined to be necessary (whether necessary or not).

From a slightly different perspective, this situation can also be seen as a three-way standoff between the patient, doctor, and the disease. The question remains: who takes the lead, and who follows the one in charge. I often refer to this situation as "who is driving the bus." Of course, there is the patient's desire for control over their own destiny, but also the healthcare practitioner's knowledge and experience which gives them an obvious advantage. The third driver is the disease or disorder itself. If the disease takes the role of the driver, both the patient and doctor are reacting to the symptoms of the disease.

This silent challenge is often the unspoken undercurrent of any initial consultation. Should we improve our understanding of the dynamics of sizing someone up, we can gain an unparalleled advantage to the psychology behind bedside manner. Recognize that as we win over a patient's trust, we become responsible for the outcome in the patient's eyes. Therefore, ethically we must treat our patients to the highest level of our ability.

When dealing with contact, we may work on a physical level, an emotional level, or both at the same time. In the physical context, we all have an idea of personal space that varies by individual, gender, and culture. In the United States, this personal space extends to just beyond arm's length. Anything outside this proximity is seen and observed, but not usually within a distance for interaction. Within this arm's length distance, there is an even closer distance approximately at elbow length that is reserved for intimate contact. Any attempt by an individual or crowd that seeks to move between these spaces rapidly without first seeking permission will be seen as threatening and aggressive. Permission to enter a space is usually given through affirmative body language and/or verbal agreement. In his book, *The Silent Language*, Edward Hall described in detail his breakdown of personal distance back in 1963. His study of "proxemics"[44] identified four distances that correspond to our "intimate," which he measured as 6–18 inches, and "personal" extending from 18 inches to 4 feet. He also described a "social" distance from 4–12 feet, at which people who are not close interact with each other. The fourth category include the "public" distance from 12– 25 feet, corresponding with public speaking/presentation interactions.

In the case of healthcare workers, mindfulness of a patient's personal and intimate distance levels will allow a more diplomatic and smooth entry into the healing interaction. As the encounter invariably begins with the physical proximity, we can then assess for the emotional contact necessary for further progress.

Verbal contact is best made with open-ended questions that allow a wide range of responses from the patient. "How are you today?" or "What seems to be the issue?" are appropriate questions, while the more specific questions may yield less information. The open nature of the question can reveal much about the person's concerns, priorities, and urgency, as well as what they do not mention but perhaps should have. Whatever information the person offers then becomes a basis for further assessment.

There is much conjecture about what allows people from varying backgrounds, ages, economic strata, and walks of life to be able to connect and have a meaningful positive relationship. The core of what makes it possible is the ability to find one or more points of commonality, that convergence of statistics and chance that two individuals coming from different directions may find something similar in their own personal history, experience, and possibly even wounding patterns. As human beings, we often look for patterns, and the individual survey points such as gender, age, ethnic group, hometown, income bracket, sports teams, and similar childhood experiences can serve to bond us in ways that make us inclusive of people who may otherwise be completely different. When we include others based on our common aspects, we are telling them that we are safe, and they are among friends as opposed to having to fend for themselves. The outward expression of "us" is another way of saying that we can join together to face against our common foes.

Consider the situation where a doctor who has hundreds of certificates mounted on the wall, multiple degrees after their name, and a long resume of highly respected institutions still occasionally has non-compliant patients. What happens in those cases that leads the patient to go their own way? I propose that the doctor is trying to engage the patient's belief system by presenting an overwhelming knowledge in science. While intellect is a celebrated criterion for belief, it is not the only currency. The unspoken assumption in modern medicine is that science is the only measure that engenders belief. If the patient values faith, humor, or life experience, the diplomas and certificates do not have the same value to them. The ability to read a patient relies on the information that they bring to the table. The greater the awareness on the part of the therapist, the more options you have to formulate your response. The ayahuasca shaman surely does not wear a white coat and have mounted diplomas in their office, yet they are perfectly capable of appealing to their clientele.

When attempting to engage a patient's belief system, we must process quickly what they have made known to us through the initial open questioning. You might think of it like being a counterpuncher in boxing. We register what is coming before quickly formulating and delivering a response. For our purposes, we engage their belief systems when we successfully connect with a subject that affirms our common interests. This reinforces the idea that we are alike and may easily share the same ideas on reasonable solutions to their problems. In effect, we are nonverbally implying that we are from the same tribe. Naturally, a doctor from the same tribe will be seen as being more responsive to a patient's concerns than someone from outside the tribe.

Conversely, when we concentrate on our differences, we separate individuals into differing groups, which emphasizes that the others will be outside the circle of familiarity and protection. This exclusion process is a common thread through our high school experiences when small groups of friends and cliques form and shift.

Specifically, if a patient comes across as an intellectual, provide them with as much information as they can handle. Include all news, relevant facts, and arguments, as well as figures that may be of interest. If a patient is driven by their faith, pray with them, or discuss similarities between your different faiths. You need not be of the same faith to pray with someone, especially if your goal is to help them heal. If the patient is independence minded, point out situations in your area of expertise that do not follow convention. Make a point of alternative therapies that may provide benefits over that of standard therapy. If the patient is humor minded, tell them a good joke that relates to their situation. If a patient endlessly complains about poor treatment from a previous doctor, respond with an emphasis on your attention to detail and insistence on not cutting corners. (At the same time, be wary that they may complain about you to their next therapist...) In the absence of all these possible avenues for connection, plain compassion for the pain, suffering, and worry of the human condition will suffice.

In emphasizing our commonalities, we can bring someone into the range of communication. When you can relate to someone due to a common experience, it is as if whispering a secret to a friend in confidence. This internal communication implies that you are working together on a common cause and reduces the natural resistance to communicating with the enemy. This is seen as safe and trustworthy, whereas talking with anyone outside the group implies exposure to danger. Any communication with the enemy must be taken with care, as you can never be sure that any message is not tinged with deception or foul play.

Once the commonality or connection is severed, the usual protective mechanisms to defend against deception are raised back up again. Recognize that this connection is vital to the smooth communication and acceptance of your offer to help and heal. Consider the image of a hand extended in friendship as a prerequisite to any patient even allowing you to come closer. This connection and contact are the surest initiator and facilitator of communication, oftentimes regardless of what is spoken afterward.

Much of our initial communication with patients relies on a simple but difficult to implement task of winning trust. Once attained, it is even more difficult to maintain over time. The idea of "saying what you do and doing what you say" is the very foundation of any type of structure that may be built. Smooth methodical movements that display your expertise and training are essential to building predictability and thus taking away any uncertainties that the patient may have brought with them. This predictability is a strong nonverbal communicator of what someone can expect from any interaction. This allays the immediate concern for most patients that you will do something that may hurt them. At the same time, any information that you can give to shed light on their illness/problem reinforces the sense of your competence. The idea of a steady hand at the wheel is our goal when we outwardly show this repetition. In fact, we are engaging the patient's subconscious mind in a training scenario where we can reinforce the ideas that bolster trustworthiness and reassurance.

Unsurprisingly, unpredictability is often associated with aggressive and dangerous behavior which negates any gains in trust that may have been established by previous healthcare professionals.

Immediately following establishment of contact and fomenting a solid connection, the next layer is that of maintaining the trust. This will rely on clearly communicating the treatment that is to be done and doing exactly what you have communicated. Avoid deception or trickery as in the old "hey, look, a bird," before quickly jabbing a child with an injection. Any betrayal of that carefully built trust may sully the hard-earned foundation gained prior to that moment.

When we consider the situation from chapter four of a personal attack against a person's container, we can see that the connection is the critical point which separates an actual attack versus someone joking with you. These personal attacks often come in the form of judgment from others as well as ridicule. A personal judgment is an attack on the container of a person, a direct attack on the choices that a person has made. Without contact and connection, any judgment is rarely seen as constructive.

One aspect that complicates our access to a patient's trust is that ridicule has been used as a method of shaping behavior for as long as we have studied psychology. It is a form of judgment that scorns a person's choices and implies that they should alter their behavior to match that of the person criticizing them. We can see this process operating as peer pressure, ridicule, and bullying. Regardless of the country or culture, our children all undergo this form of behavioral modification on a daily basis to different degrees. In extreme cases, the ridicule becomes bullying, especially when developing children are unknowingly reacting to other negative influences in their lives.

Should we insert a connection and contact into the aforementioned attack, it is more likely to be seen as a joke or something constructive for the purpose of teaching. It is the manner by which we pass on our individual culture, family traditions, and general teaching. One common form of contact is showing that you care about the person. The love and caring are necessary to establish a nonthreatening motive. As a healthcare professional, caring is the critical bridge that allows us to get across to any wounded individual.

In considering "social distancing" as devised during pandemic situations, the connections that we establish will be at a social distance until the point of treatment and physical contact. This emphasizes the need to have a strong connection prior to actual treatment as the usual feeling-out period may be compressed. Your efforts at building the connection are not diminished, even if separated by a mask, plexiglass screen, or computer monitor. Consistency in both verbal communication and body language will always be vital to continue the trust that eliminates unpleasant surprises.

CHAPTER 9

The Bedside Manner Toolbox

The maxim of "laughter is the best medicine" applies to the use of humor in blunting the impact of unexpected or unwanted information with regard to health. Scientifically speaking, humor is the combination of the detection of an incongruent concept (something that doesn't match up with expectations), the emotional response, and then the activation of the reward systems in the brain.[45] The discussion of what constitutes as effective humor will lie outside the scope of our current discourse. Nevertheless, when we poke fun at ourselves or particular human conditions, we are drawing a connection between ourselves and the patient. We are essentially using humor as the contact that allows you to approach and come into a closer social distance for interaction. These non-directed jokes are the best types of humor to utilize, as it is serving as the critical contact for delivering sobering news. This contact will limit or even prevent the alienation of the patient and emphasize the caring and empathy bond. Although popular, humor that belittles or denigrates should be avoided in these instances. When effective humor is utilized, we are imprinting the association of the experience with us and connecting it directly to the reward pathways in the brain.[46] This process can be very powerful as you are literally rewiring a person to feel a reward whenever you tell a good joke.[47] Used in combination with proper treatment, it is easy to envision use of this tool to effect positive behavioral changes to ingrain healthy habits. (A little biscuit for good behavior, anyone?)

Distractions are another way of diverting the immediate attention of a patient away from anxiety or an otherwise uncomfortable situation. In essence, it can decoy the patient away from feeding energy into an undesirable outcome. As the anxiety comes from a place of insecurity of a negative outcome or impending pain, turning their attention to something that reminds them of a pleasant experience may be helpful. Clues as to possible topics may be found in the choice of clothing, reading material, brand of car keys, or anything that has been expressed as a hobby or favorite pastime.

Keep in mind that humor can also be used as a distraction. The timing of the humor is particularly important as it serves as an excellent ice-breaker but can become an impediment if it keeps you from progressing in your chosen treatment plan. Just the right amount of humor to break the tension of anxiety and then to relate to a topic that may be a shared interest (i.e. cooking, fishing, travel, hiking) may be enough to relax a person enough to allow a smoother course of treatment. Even friendly banter will distract the patient from the expectations of pain. Conversations with specific themes will also engage the left brain and will divert their attention away from the inevitable negative repetitive ruminations.

While humor and distractions can ease the transitions, clear communication and preceding each step with expression of appropriate expectations will go a long way toward easing the discomfort of an otherwise awkward social situation. If we can actively employ this coping mechanism to deal with anticipated stress and introduce humor and laughter as a way of preempting an overly serious situation, our ability to discuss a range of issues widens.

When patients resort to humor, it is critical to see their humor as their coping mechanism for anxiety. In fact, it is possibly the most common effective coping mechanism for tense or sober talk. If we can identify the attempted humor (whether it is actually funny, is another story) as their coping process, we will see that it doesn't necessarily require a response. Merely listening to the joke is enough to create a bond.

In instances where there is some ambiguity as to whether a connection is made, it helps to lead with sympathy or empathy. I remember once watching a Brene Brown animated short film where she compares *sympathy* to *empathy*. The *sympathy* was portrayed by a cute animal character standing at the rim of a large hole looking down at a second animal character sitting inside the hole. He smugly asks if the character inside the hole would like a sandwich. For *empathy*, we see a ladder propped from the rim to the bottom of the hole and both animal characters looking up from inside the hole together.

When we deliver "bad" news, we will need to employ both sympathy and empathy. Sympathy guides the approach and depending on the needs of the patient, we can either engage with deeper empathy (more contact) or disengage altogether (less contact). Going by feel allows you to sense the needs of the patient based on their body or verbal language. Most people will give you some idea of which way they are feeling prior to explicitly telling you so. Some patients will need contact and in these instances, we will need to respond with empathy. Gentle non-threatening physical contact and a show of concern are both forms of soothing behavior. Expressions of personal experience regarding the feelings involved bring everything closer to home. This may also initiate a conversation with the patient that allows them to express their feelings without judgment. Affirmation and listening can be extremely therapeutic in these situations.

For those that require space and freedom to reassess their situation and just think, sympathy is necessary. When a person is overwhelmed and is seeking space, any further contact can be seen as threatening. Limiting the contact to the equivalent of an arm's-length pat on the shoulder may be all that is warranted. Most people can discern between an expression of genuine feeling versus just an attempt at being polite. Giving space allows someone who is overwhelmed time to sort their thoughts and feelings. Despite attempts to the contrary, there is no automated robot at this point that can deliver either of these intrinsically organic levels of contact and connection.

CHAPTER 10

Memory, Sensitivity, *and* the Coping Threshold

When we consider the situations under which a patient seeks medical help, anxiety seems to be a common thread. The underlying nervousness does also seem to influence how the brain records memory. It seems that self-described high anxiety subjects (80 undergraduate psychology students at University of Waterloo, Canada) who were exposed to negative images (pictures of accidents, people suffering, or acts of violence), had significantly better accuracy in recall of words printed next to the pictures.[48] The accuracy returned to baseline when neutral pictures (objects with no emotional attachment, e.g. a house, ship, or a chair) were used. However, there is a significant downside to this memory as it is often tainted with negative feelings which can be even further reinforced by the context of a "bad day."

While we can surmise that this phenomenon may be helpful to avoid dangerous situations for basic survival, it can also be a disincentive to seeking medical care. The stress of "white coat syndrome," where patients routinely have higher blood pressures when in the environment of a medical facility, is very real. It is useful to anyone working in a medical setting that a patient's memory of their visit may be subject to their disposition on the day in question. Practically speaking, consider a patient who slept through their morning alarm, was stuck in traffic and yelled at by their boss, and then came to your office. Regardless of what happened during the appointment, the patient's negative mindset may tint your conversation in their memory as rude or even confrontational. On the other hand, they may remember the factual details of the appointment very well.

With these caveats in mind, we can begin to see how each person's perspective may be colored based on the context of events that happen before. These peculiarities of evolution remain in our psychology and can significantly affect our ability to communicate with patients. We may never register that scary music during a television program about surgical disasters may be deeply embedded in a person's psyche, thus stunting our ability to reach out to help them. Our media is rife with examples of negative headlines subtly yet purposely placed next to pictures of people to subconsciously link the two. The manipulation of this very phenomenon by politicians has proven extremely effective in shaping the perceptions of individuals up to entire populations. By grouping people or actions into a positive or negative context, the human memory can be influenced to specific ends. The very neurological machinery that records a single memory is subject to many steps of interpretation. It is remarkable that it even works to the speed and efficiency to which we are accustomed.

In 1991, psychologist and author Elaine Aron introduced the idea of the Highly Sensitive Person (HSP)[49], allowing us to input another crucial concept in our overall map of the patient psyche. She describes the idea that people have varying sensitivities to external stimulus, be it through any of our five common senses. She notes that her research reveals approximately 20% of humanity belongs to a group that has a heightened sensitivity to all stimuli but lower threshold to being overwhelmed. Conversely, there is another 20% who have a low sensitivity, but a very high threshold to feeling inundated and stressed out. The remaining 60% of the population lies somewhere in between these extremes. While Aron has done extensive work on the HSP, it is the concept of external stimulus that I found most applicable to my model.

I find that every patient arrives with a baseline level of stimulation in their lives. This may come in the form of unruly children, traffic, work stresses, pain from a medical condition, or emotional pain from a trau-matic social situation. We are generally able to cope with most of these stresses and will function normally in our lives on a day-to-day basis. However, as Aron and others have found, there is a limit to what we can handle in our conscious mind (that is, the left and right brain). We will call this limit the "coping threshold." Beyond this limit, behavior may become erratic, with incremental loss of normal control of the conscious mind. These stresses over long term can be programmed into the sub-conscious mind, and we see secondary effects of previous trauma such as developed phobias and patterns of aversions to anything that may remind the patient of the original trauma. It appears that the trauma response can also be inadvertently trained. In other words, the repeated exposure to phobias conditions the nerve pathways to the amygdala, the affected area of the brain in control of the fight-or-flight response.[50] Every subsequent exposure to the phobia trains the response to occur with increasing speed and efficiency. Fortunately, the human body and mind are capable of healing from most of these deep-set traumas.

The matter at hand, however, is that all humans have a point after which we can all become overwhelmed.[51] This point varies in different people and also depends on the timing. Each patient already brings with them their baseline level of stimulation prior to our assessment of their condition, and we need to take this into account. When any patient is already overwhelmed, this may significantly affect our success in treating their condition. For example, if the patient had to fight through heavy traffic just to reach their appointment time with you, they may have phys-iologically measurable increases in breathing rate and blood pressure. I have observed in my practice the decrease in pain threshold (thus greater post-treatment pain) when dealing with an already overwhelmed patient. Thus one of the primary assessments at that first appointment will be to determine where the limit to the patient's normal coping systems lies. A line of questioning to this end can be casually included into any initial greeting ("How are you feeling today?" or "Do you have a lot on your plate right now?") and continued by addressing their answer directly.

A number of years ago, one patient, Claire, presented to an initial consultation twenty minutes late carrying multiple bags from shopping and complaining of heavy traffic and difficulty finding a parking spot. She was breathing heavily and her hair looked disheveled. She was dropping items out of her bags, then picking them up haphazardly. During the course of our consultation, I sought to determine her baseline level of stress while trying to estimate her ability to cope with her existing stresses. She happened to be very well educated with a tremendous coping mechanism, but her plate was mostly full already that day.

Typically, for Claire's intelligence level, I would have described her current condition along with the proposed treatment plan in great detail to satisfy her need for information. In this instance, considering her nearly loaded coping mechanisms, I elected to gently reduce the information load (fewer details with limited bullet points) and deal with emotional stress as a priority. Australian psychologist John Sweller introduced his Cognitive Load Theory in 1988,[52] which noted that everyone has a certain amount of "working memory" which is distinct from short-term and long-term memory. Should this working memory be occupied with non-essential information (distractions or things that stress you out), then further capacity is limited. Instead of overwhelming her with detailed information, we discussed the base emotions that she was feeling and how she managed to keep everything so "well balanced." Of course, this was a bit of a prod to get her to discuss her active effort at coping with her stresses. I delivered her treatment plan in segments, concentrating on taking one step at a time. It is safe to say that as fatigue sets in, the intellectual abilities wane. With this temporary decline, patients adjust and rely more on their base emotions to get by until they are able to rest and refresh. Eventually, she still sought the detailed information, but I waited on her cue to address it directly. As it happened, she was able to adapt her coping mechanism to include the stresses from the consultation and impending treatment.

These traumas, including physical, emotional, and perceived stresses, all accumulate over a period of time. Fortunately, there is a built-in decay rate associated with short-term memory loss. The observed decay of memory over time serves as a self-healing method employed by the body to assist in the healing process of accumulated traumas. In neurological terms, the transfer of the non-salient short-term working memory (stored in the hippocampus) into the long-term episodic and semantic memory (encoded into the cortex) is disabled by selective culling in the consolidation stage. It has been noted that sleep enhances both consolidation of memories as well as forgetting.[53] Conversely, children that cannot forget childhood trauma develop significant neurobiological disorders throughout life (Teicher and Samson, 2016, citation 30).

The net damage suffered becomes the accumulated quantity of traumas minus the time it takes for the memory of that trauma to dull. There has been much speculation and observation on this front over decades.[54] Therefore, great care must be taken for any person to reduce the regular trauma to below the rate of memory decay in order to maintain a healthy balance. It is unclear whether cumulative damage over a lifetime can be reversed, but unchecked damage from specific stresses has been studied. In a 35-year longitudinal population study, Johansson et al.[55] found an association between the amount of psychological stress in middle-aged women and the future development of dementia. The 1,462 women in the study who reported frequent or constant stress during the any of the examinations had a significantly higher rate of Alzheimer's disease, vascular dementia, and other types of dementia. Deleterious effects of stress that exceeded the coping capacity had been noted in cases of soldiers suffering from "trench mouth" during the first World War. In these cases, prolonged stress (the risk and fear of impending severe injury or death) led to the direct suppression of the immune system and subsequent severe oral infection. Another more recent study in mice noted the effect of stress as induced by pain on the increase of gray hair.[56]

Another point that I cannot emphasize enough is the need for all healthcare practitioners to assess patient urgency based on their coping capacity. Questions regarding how a person deals with stress need to be asked early in the assessment stage. The effectiveness of their methods bears a great deal of importance on reduction of chronic damage over time. An emergency to some patients may not necessarily rise to the level of an emergency to the nurse or doctor relative to other patients. Obviously, any given patient's urgency may not necessarily be realistic ("I want this done yesterday!") given rational expectations for treatment times and the practical availability of each person treating them (i.e., the doctor is booked until next Tuesday). While every attempt can be made to match the patient urgency with appropriate treatment timetables, we can also alter the patient expectations with education and active reorganization of their treatment plans. Assessment of the coping capacity will also give hints as to the amount of psychological support necessary to ensure a positive patient experience.

Any discussion of stress and trauma in our patients would be incomplete without tackling an important question most of us have faced at one time or another: With increasing recognition of mental diseases, when should a healthcare professional contemplate a referral to a psychological and/or psychiatric specialist? Considering our developing concept of emotional balance, the idea of mental health has a fair-sized gray zone. Where do we delineate between disease and the diversity of the normal everyday state? Taking this diversity of what can be considered normal into account, we must look at the basic function of mental health as a component of general health. As a clinician who primarily deals with the public, I have seen a wide range of people who range from robust mental health to visibly mentally impaired. In addition, there is now increasing awareness of the wide range of autistic spectrum that was not previously available. The communication through body language is every bit as important as that which is communicated verbally. In many instances, the two tracks will tell entirely different stories. While this is clearly a red flag, the pertinent question arises of what we consider to be something that reaches a threshold of referral to a mental health specialist.

In examining our parameters, the main concern is a deleterious condition that is either of extreme severity or of long duration. Signs of overwhelmed coping mechanisms are key to this assessment. What is the patient's threshold, and where are they in relation to their limits? Symptoms that impair a maintainable steady state are key points for inspection. The perspective taken by the patient is critical, and the idea of rebalancing an aspect that we can clearly observe can be a way of reducing the severity of the problem. As a whole, any manifestation of severe imbalance that exceeds the patient's coping capacity is a primary reason for referral to a mental health specialist. Any debilitation in caring for oneself as an individual that lasts for more than one month is also a major indicator for referral.

In the context of bedside manner, our goal is to better connect and communicate with our patients. There is a current standard of care for the specialties of medicine and dentistry that has been established over time and much effort by many dedicated and talented individuals. Consider that our observations may be the first step in getting help to those that need specialized care. In delving deeply into the psyche, we gain much insight into many of the problems that develop from miscommunications between our conscious and subconscious minds. In our capacity as health practitioners, we have few opportunities to affect traumas that have lingered over a lifetime. One step at a time, we may be able to make substantive changes collectively, either through our own treatment programs or by connecting our patients with specialists that can help to improve their mental health.

CHAPTER 11

Building *the* Doctor-Patient Relationship

O ne key aspect of the communication between the patient and doctor must be the expectation of the type of relationship—the expectation of a short-term vs. a long-term relationship. There are many patients who view health and treatment in a transactional manner. In other words, they believe they are buying a product which may or may not come with a warranty. They do so in the belief that the treatment is a simple affair of taking a pill which will cure the disease. It is quite possible that the allopathic medicine model was so effective in marketing that many patients still see this as the only way that medicine works: take a medicine, cure the disease. This is akin to purchasing a cream at a pharmacy that relieves itching. They may apply the cream at their own discretion, requiring very little to no further discussion or guidance. It is also with the expectation that there is nothing more severe that they will need to address. They also do this in the interest of saving money as well as retaining control in deciding if they want to partake in parts of the treatment that may be unpalatable, i.e., painful, inconvenient in timing, or distasteful in some other manner. In some cases, this may be adequate, but in the case of many chronic conditions, it is quite insufficient for effecting the changes in behavior necessary to shift a major imbalance (such as managing diabetes).

The other end of the spectrum to a short-term transactional relationship is the long-term management relationship. For disorders such as periodontal disease and diabetes, regular management and feedback is as vital as the initial treatment itself. For example, if you are brushing your teeth incompletely or incorrectly, you will naturally have areas that you miss. These areas will eventually build up plaque and tartar, thus changing the overall bacterial profile in your mouth. After approximately three weeks, the tartar hardens, you will be unable to remove the deposits with a toothbrush or any other home hygiene implement. Thus, is it imperative that you remove the softer plaque with brush and floss prior to it becoming so calcified that it becomes clinically impossible to remove without metal and ultrasonic instruments. If you get the necessary feedback regarding the areas you are missing, you will be less likely to pass the point where tartar buildup is impossible to remove without heavy equipment. Regular feedback and daily care become paramount to the treatment of the disease.

There is a widespread misunderstanding involved in all types of medicine where patients shop for prices. Especially in highly competitive marketplaces, the belief that they are buying a product was instilled deeply in much of our population. While there are some treatments where this model may work, there are others where it is deeply misrepresented. Case in point: dental implants. While it is often times seen as a product where you can effectively compare prices charged by different doctors, it is a much more complicated affair that deserves further examination. In my humble opinion, a dental implant is one of the longer-term relationships that is possible. The reasoning is that while the implant industry success rate is excellent, the regular care of the implant is vital to the long-term survivability. The fact that the patient lost that particular tooth is accompanied by the susceptibility that caused the tooth loss. In other words, there was some reason that specific tooth was lost as opposed to other teeth that were retained. Did that particular tooth have a cavity, periodontal disease, bone loss, or a split in the root that made it harder to clean? Did this patient grind their teeth with a premature contact on this particular tooth? If any of the answers to these questions are in the affirmative, we may presume that the implant will also be subjected to the same susceptibilities. When these variables are in play, it becomes critical to have a dentist who understands them and regularly monitors these parameters. A patient who is not aware that these problems exist will be thoroughly ignorant of the care necessary to prevent them. Thus when we truly understand the differences between the short- and long-term relationships necessary, we can ensure that the patient expectations are appropriate with their actual needs. This is a key aspect of the communication that must be established for effective and successful care and treatment. Patients may find that they really need the long-term relationship to make their treatment successful and perform as they expected for many years.

As the patient expectations vary, the practitioner will need to improvise their approach towards a patient's initial stance. It would be appropriate to address the patient's short-term need and then discuss the importance of long-term care. Of course, we have no real control over extenuating circumstances in the patient's life yet imprinting the need for a long-term plan does plant the seed for a more comprehensive relationship.

Another basic concept in our mental map will consist of the conflicting ideas of structure versus freedom. One example is teaching painting in an art class. The structured approach is a step-by-step tutorial to emphasize the styles and methods to achieve the desired final product. The other end of the spectrum is akin to giving the artist a set of parameters for a painting and then allowing them to create their interpretation. Both seek to achieve a similar goal, but the amount of support given to each student will depend on their personalities, experience, and confidence. These are both valid teaching methods and represent the difference between a step-by-step prescribed method of intellectual learning (structure), versus a creative approach, which allows a person to free form a solution to a given problem (freedom). These are two fundamental approaches to how the mind builds understanding in any subject. As such, the cues that a patient offers will inform you of their preference in how they learn.

For example, a patient who seeks structure in learning about a disease may ask about the specifics on how a genetic mutation affects the cells, with the change in key protein configurations, leading to the physical manifestations of the disease. A way to satisfy this need for structure would be offering a detailed description of the signs and symptoms then increasing in detail as necessary. You may need to explicitly state the cause of the disease and itemize the goals of a method of treatment. Once that structure has been satisfied, the patient will indicate an understanding of the subject and for you to stop increasing the details.

It is particularly noteworthy that a person seeking structure is looking to intellectually grasp a usually complex set of ideas in a short period of time. Simplifying professional terminology to layman's speech will assist greatly in your ultimate goal of education and establishing the structure. Recognize that whenever someone asks, "What's the plan," they are asking you to provide the structure for them to bridge the gap in their understanding. In a vacuum of intellectual structure, they cannot move forward without knowing what you intend to do to solve their problem. For these patients who need guidance, speaking from a position of an instructor or that of a senior helps support their expectations of your role. It is in these instances that the "white coat" of a doctor or therapist can actively improve patient compliance. Fortunately for most medical professionals, the idea of a treatment plan is quite familiar and should not present much of an obstacle.

The need for freedom is seen in situations where a patient seeks multiple options but does not ask many detail questions. When we encounter this lack of interest in the details, there is a likely orientation toward "feel." They are not so much encumbered by the specifics of the treatment but whether they can trust you to be sensitive to their needs. Trust is elevated to the highest priority, and every time that you tell them what to expect and it comes to pass, their trust in you is reinforced. They may be undecided on their course of treatment and will sometimes have difficulty choosing between divergent options. Perhaps contrary to their best interests, many patients in this category seek inordinate opinions from people within their circle of trust (some of whom have no particular expertise in the field) and ultimately decide on a direction based on consensus as well as how it feels. Many will often want to chart their own course through treatment and wish to be given all possible options. However, what they truly seek is for someone to take care of the details and customize a plan that addresses their priorities. Note that a patient exhibiting a tendency toward "freedom" may not respond as well to directives and orders. They are more likely to accept an "eye-level" approach in which you relate to them as a peer rather than dictate to them as a superior.

Recognizing this dichotomy will allow you to feed the mind of the patient in a mutually satisfying manner such that proper treatment may be rendered. There will also be combinations of the two in different proportions. They could be equally important to a patient, so you will need to establish their priority list. The method you use to frame the options will and should be customized to how the patient hears you. Rather than telling them what they want to hear, the observant healthcare practitioner gives them the information they need in the manner that they need to receive it.

CHAPTER 12

Conscious vs Subconscious Decision-Making

Consider the range of processes which lead up to major decisions in not only healthcare but life in general. Conscious decision-making centers on the concept of the left and right brain dominance. With left brain dominance, there is an intellectually minded decision-making process which leans on reason and logic, carefully considering benefits versus disadvantages, cost versus benefit, and perceived length of healing time (or time off work). On the other end of the spectrum is an emotional-based process involving how much the final result will appeal to the patient's idea of improvement, the perceived gains in esthetics, the associated side benefits of treatment, along with the perceived physical pain of healing. Often, patients of this type will bring a photograph of how they want to look after a given procedure. We can describe these processes as the classic "right and left brain" contrast. There is also a myriad of combinations of the two extremes with an ocean of possibilities in between. If we as therapists are able to sort out the motivations underlying our patients' decisions, we would be in a better position to support our patients when they inevitably ask, "What would you do in my situation?" One tricky aspect will be the direction from which they approach the problem.

Is the approach from a position of an actively empowered person determined to solve the problem despite facing an overwhelming situation or that of a passive victim who will ultimately succumb to the negative effects of the disease? The primary difference lies in the refusal of the empowered person to accept the negative circumstance as a permanent feature. The negative situation is in turn used to fuel a positive response that allows the patient to change of balance of their disease and seek the treatment they need. In contrast, the victim mentality delays the patient from actively getting the treatment they need and allowing the accumulation of "damage" to continue unabated. The idea of a self-fulfilling prophecy comes to mind in the situation of the victim due to the inability to properly respond to a disease challenge.

What is the deciding factor that truly triggers a person to use the full force of their abilities to face a medical problem (or other type of major issue)? Once again, for some it is the accumulation of a critical mass of information which leads to an internal momentum (subconscious mind) from which a patient can move. In feeding their lack of information with facts, figures, studies, and success/failure rates, you may feed the intellectual left brain. For others, the decision to face a problem is a right-brain emotional one from which one will need to fully digest the mental impact of the disease upon the host. Once the feeling of pain and loss is fully felt, only then can the person convert the negatives of the disease into the ultimate positive decision to actively live. This living within the feeling is necessary for the next step which is to find the missing element that will help them deal with their immediate medical problem. This is where empathy and understanding without pressure will once again feed the subconscious mind to respond. Ultimately, we want the patient to seek the expert with the awareness of the disease, experience in dealing with the treatment and aftermath, and the willingness to listen to how they are feeling. In both appealing to the left-brain intellect as well as to the right-brain emotion, we need to feed the subconscious while still satisfying the immediate needs of the left and the right brains.

It has been my personal experience that while an intellectual approach is often viewed as the main driver, most major decisions are made through the emotions and feelings. This realization places the area of mind activity directly into the subconscious. As stated before, the subconscious mind collects information constantly and subtly— and often below the threshold of a bullet point. It records information until it sorts out the salient core which is what eventually is sent to our conscious mind. Therefore, it includes physical details that allow us to "picture" the context of an activity or event as well as the exact minutia of the thinking during the event. When we consider the source of this gut feeling as a subconscious communication, we find that people gravitate toward the external sources of whatever they themselves are missing. In other words, the subconscious directs the person to seek what they need to make itself whole again.

We must consider that while the intellect guides us, the subconscious is what pushes us to follow through with the chosen path as directed or stop us from proceeding with a gut feeling.

Subconscious decision-making is akin to autopilot. It is composed of the collection of skills, knowledge, and habits learned over time. When we are not actively engaged in thinking about a subject or activity, our subconscious is making the decisions for us by way of communication through feeling. Left to a patient's own devices, they will gravitate towards what feels right to them.

This idea of feeling right deserves closer examination as it involves a person's evolutionarily vital desire for existence. It is safe to say that the human mind and body do whatever is necessary for its own survival. If it is cold, our bodies shiver to create warmth. If we touch a flame, we recoil our hands to avoid it. Outside the conscious realm, the subconscious directs all humans to automatically react to a negative stimulus by escaping from the stimulus. It then creates a negative memory proportional to the perceived danger of the episode.

This action/reaction response to various stimuli is not only present for the most basic survival mechanisms such as body temperature regulation or immune response to a bacteria or virus. We repeatedly see this snap reaction response in the emotions that guide the subconscious mind to avoid any perceived pain.

In observing the body's response to a disease stimulus, we need only look at the activity of coronavirus in the 2002–2003 SARS and the COVID-19 pandemic. Many of the fatalities were due to a phenomenon called "cytokine storm." In certain patients, the viral impact on the lungs led to a systemic reaction by the immune system, releasing massive amounts of cytokines, chemicals that normally trigger inflammation and a defensive immune response. Rather than a measured response to the virus, the overreaction of full body cytokine release created such a massive inflammation event that it resulted in multiple organ failure. When we come to see the mechanics of the action and reaction, it provides us entry points to prevent the ultimate negative result: patient mortality.

Time and time again, we can witness the actions and reactions that govern many processes in biology, chemistry, physics, medicine, human psychology, and societies in general. At each step, there is a possibility of inappropriate or outsized reactions to the initial insult stimulus. In other words, a patient's perception of pain during their experience has everything to do with whether their memory distorts it into a massive ordeal or deemphasizes it as one memory among many. This holds true within the psyche of any individual and the process by which life decisions are made.

Some of the actions we take are fueled by internal desires, and result in truly original output that reflects our unique character. These types of actions can be initiated through the intellectual left brain as well as the creative right brain, or both at the same time.

Many of our daily actions, however, are simply reactions to external forces. For example, if someone calls you a weakling, one possible response is to show that you are not weak by regularly going to the gym. Another example involving health is a doctor telling you that you have Type 2 diabetes. Your reaction may include exercising, weight loss, watching your diet, and careful blood glucose monitoring. While our populace and healthcare system in the United States is keenly aware of the need to actively seek healthy choices and balance, most of what brings patients to seek medical care is still reactionary.

On the negative side, a person may react to excessive stress through tobacco, alcohol, marijuana, or overeating. Many of these reactions can become habits if they are even mildly successful in relief of stress. Self-activating triggered programs within the subconscious mind dominate much of our reactions.

The parts of the brain that engage are often dependent upon whether we see any action or reaction as a single event or linked to a greater pattern. For these single events of action and reaction, the intellectual left brain usually remains dominant, although the emotional right brain can be mildly involved. The ability to remain rational in the face of a single insult is highly likely. For instance, imagine standing in line at the supermarket. When you casually look at the magazines, someone cuts the line in front of you. You will follow a process of decision-making to address the action of the instigator. Much of our ability to problem solve involves our ability to react in a timely and appropriate manner. Indeed, this ability to solve presented problems is often used as a gauge of intelligence in many study models. Reactions to these types of single events typically remain measured and muted, as the offense is limited to a one-time event. The tendency to be able to dismiss it and blow it off is more likely.

If your mind recognizes the event as the beginning of a pattern (multiple transgressions that begin to highlight a negative trend) and not just an isolated occurrence, we start to see the right-brain emotional response rise to equal the original left-brain activity. There is an evaluation period when both left and right brains are equally engaged, awaiting the final trigger for a trained response. We begin to think about what to do in the event "another bastard cuts us in line." The intellectual response is retained, but there is an addition of more emotion into the equation. There is often an associated feeling of injury which persists to begin programing of the subconscious mind.

When the offense is part of a long-standing pattern, we start to see the subconscious now take a dominant role, particularly if you notice the same person repeatedly cut others in line over an extended period of time. The emotional insult of the person cutting the line again becomes too great to ignore. The subconscious pent-up anger of previous transgressions combines with the current situation and demands a response to stop any further offense. As the seat of long-term learning, we find that previous responses that were successful will be trained into subconscious memory, and every subsequent hint of the same pattern will be met with a more rapid response. Especially if the pattern is well known, a trained response becomes automatic. Whether we then decide to verbally engage the line cutter, kick them out of line, or engage in fisticuffs, it will depend on whatever is effective.

When relating back to patient care, careful observation will reveal whether they are engaged in a negative cycle of reaction to previous people or experiences. Are you experiencing significant patient pushback or an active avoidance of a therapy that you know to be helpful? Is there a phobia or a latent fear that needs addressing? There is constant interplay between the conscious and the subconscious that varies within a person when making major health decisions. Redirecting their energy towards fulfilling their true fundamental needs will bring them out of their repeating cycles and reset their path towards a more fulfilling goal.

While reading body language is important to assess the disposition of the patient, a healthcare practitioner can actually change the direction of that interaction to project the desired outcome for the patient. In other words, by projecting their own body language associated with a "successful" outcome, a healthcare practitioner can affect the patient to believe that the likelihood of a positive outcome is inevitable. This reduces the impact of a result hinging on the success or failure of any singular aspect of the treatment. In doing so, we can use the placebo effect to our advantage as the patient will improve their own chances of success through stimulated activation of their own healing response and immune system. Be mindful to emphasize the positive body language but avoid unattainable promises verbally. Trust can be easily broken irretrievably by over-promising and under-delivering.

This manner of telling yourself a successful story to enliven the image of your goal is not a new technique in psychology and is often called *cognitive reframing*. Simply put, it is replacing negative thoughts with positive ones, turning previous hopelessness into new possibilities. This technique allows you restate a goal on a daily basis such that you open or widen the possibility in your mind that a seemingly far-fetched goal will become reachable. This affirmation sets a baseline from which you can start to measure progress and thus create a momentum which finally pushes your subconscious into action.

In the case of a healer and/or medical practitioner, you are in a position to change the storyline of the goal to affect a successful outcome, whether it is smoking cessation, dental rehabilitation, or a hip replacement surgery. Unlike the popular "The Law of Attraction,"[57] which postulates that we can manifest things into our personal lives by intention, we as healthcare professionals are in a position to divert psychological belief for our patient's benefit. The idea of "like attracts like" has been discussed extensively in various healing and spiritual traditions and has its share of devotees. For our purposes, we can employ the psychology behind it to recruit any possible advantage for healing. As you change this narrative for the benefit of the patient, you can set different types of goals from short-term to longer-term goals over time. These will create structure for the patient to reach a final destination of an ultimate goal of full recovery. One must take care to create reachable goals to begin the process, as there is no inertia at the start.

Multiple studies of hip replacement surgery outcomes have found that the attitude of a patient has a great deal to do with the eventual adaptation and success rates of the replacement hip.[58] The perceived amount of pain experienced by post-surgical patients are significantly reduced with simple optimism.[59] Patients have a profound effect on their own ability to adapt and heal based on their belief system.[60] As such, if we as doctors and healthcare practitioners can access and activate this basic human response to improve our chances of success, it becomes more than just being cheerful or positive. Engaging both verbal cues ("when you recover," as opposed to "if") and body language, we can impart this outlook onto those that we treat.

Keep in mind that projecting the body language associated with success does not mean that we are promising or guaranteeing an outcome. It is simply showing through nonverbal means how it could look like in the event of a complete smashing success. We in turn as healthcare providers must believe that our treatments will improve the situation and ensure that we do not inadvertently signal our doubts to the treatment recipient. It is our challenge to envision the appearance of success and be able to channel that positive vibe to every discussion in which we engage with our patients.

The idea of envisioning and manifesting a desired result may sound like reading Rhonda Byrne's *The Secret*[61] too many times, but there is an underlying practical reason for its popularity to many devoted followers. Many of us have grown up without fully understanding our ego and sense of personal worth. People the world over tend to gauge their personal self-worth on their successes and failures in selected tasks. When we have a losing streak, we feel depressed and unworthy. On a winning streak, we feel like we're on top of the world.

This linking of success with self-worth is not a new idea. However, there is a less visible effect of this phenomenon. Many individuals steer their life choices based on what will allow them to win, thus feeding their ego. This is one popular subconscious method of choosing a career. This invariably ties their self-worth to their job and career.

We tend to choose what we are good at rather than something we love. This is exactly the reason why many recent retirees lose their sense of self-worth right after retirement and miss the feeling of regularly engaging in an activity at which they developed an expertise and allowed them to succeed. The absence of being good at something directly tied to their ego is felt more than the actual love of the job itself. Recent retirees often lapse into depression unless they commence another activity that replaces the missing elements. Subconsciously, we tend not to choose things at which we feel we are not good or will lead to eventual failure. When we take a closer look at these choices, we can see that there is an internal judgment that decides to tackle challenges in life based on the likelihood of success. I suspect our own choices may read like a laundry list of items that match up with what our egos needed at the time.

When we envision a possible future, we are engaging our imaginations to create something that does not yet exist. The main point of this statement is that we are creating a blueprint and structure necessary for future development. In short, we are laying out plans for a goal. This structure and plan significantly increase our chances of success in the chosen endeavor. As such, we are actually programming our minds to bring about the success that we have envisioned. Others see our plan for success and are attracted to us by the same mechanism that seeks to feed the ego by choosing things that allow them to succeed and thus improve their self-esteem.

While this may seem like an indictment of the egocentrically driven, this process is not to be judged as good or bad. It is nothing more or less than a basic building block of the psyches of all human beings. The ego is essential to our sense of self and critical to a healthy mental and physical steady state. When relating to our healthcare, the health professional with the plan that matches the patient's idea of success becomes the obvious choice. However, we must listen to and read the patient to best evaluate their idea of success.

CHAPTER 13

Defeating *the* Behaviors *that* Work Against Us

Once we have established a general treatment plan that addresses the patient's chief concerns, we are on our way towards our goal of health. The quality and execution of that plan serves as a foundational brick upon which the patient can further build. With every perceived success, we are guiding our patients to a place of strong belief in our teamwork. However, the treatment plan only returns the patient back to a physical whole or reasonable facsimile. Taking into account the patient's unconscious reactions, built-in coping mechanisms, self-defeating feedback loops, and other personal limitations, our treatment is doomed to failure if we do not address the factors that made the patient susceptible to disease in the first place.

Let us refer back to our patient Ella. After detailed conversation and observation established Ella's medical and dental history, it was clear that her past had quite an impact on her current conditions. Recognition of the love she shared with her mother was a logical starting point, as it allowed us to bridge the gap between the youthful, beautiful teenager with which she still identified and the aged, tired version sitting before us. Seeing her as the person she had wanted to be and engaging in our conversation in that light showed her that we too can glimpse through her eyes. In doing so, we acknowledged that her current struggles are but temporary obstacles to regaining what she used to love about herself. We also concentrated on the love shown by her two daughters in the form of financial help for her medical bills.

In arranging our appointments around her busy church attendance, we worked her scheduling around her major priorities. Just prior to commencing active treatment, we prayed together to ask for strength, guidance, and a quick recovery. This engagement of her belief system aided tremendously in her compliance with taking antibiotics, anti-inflammatories, and postoperative instructions. Her positive attitude and willingness to adhere to recommendations were quite welcome and likely decreased her postoperative soreness as well as improved her healing. During Ella's extended visits, we not only served as her periodontist but also her counselor, health guide, and eventually friend.

On the whole, we need to ask the question of whether Ella's inadequate home care was a reaction to poor communication within her marriages. Is she likely to be successful in our treatment but backslide due to personality tendencies? Does her life scarring make her more susceptible to relapse? Completion of her treatment appears to have only been a short-term goal. Ultimately, we return to the idea of balance as our long-term destination.

PART 3

Establishing and Maintaining Balance

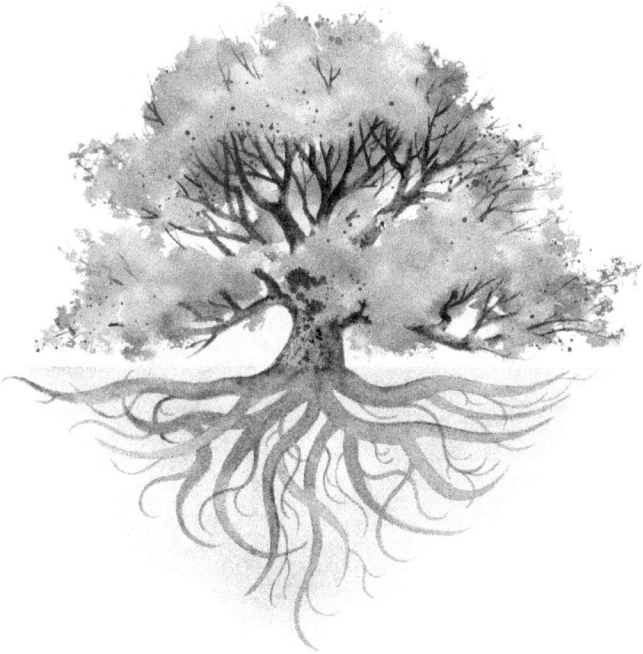

When we examine the meaning of *healing*, the most succinct definition of the term is found in Merriam-Webster: "to make free from injury or disease: to make sound or whole."[62] With this definition in mind, it depends on the idea of what constitutes "whole." While the first interpretation directly involves an injury or disease, it is clearly from the allopathic medicine model where an individual is considered healthy if they do not have an injury or known disease. This assumes that the normal steady state prior to injury or disease is optimal health. In the experience of myself and many others, this model is inadequate in many cases of chronic conditions that deal with imbalances in the body or long-term management of aging, and wear/tear issues. The latter part of this definition also deals with the idea of self and what constitutes "sound or whole." This is precisely the reason that we need to consider the variabilities in the idea of "whole." Each potential patient will arrive with a different idea of their baseline for health. Finding that baseline will allow the proper communication to commence.

Over the years, I have inherently sought balance in my own life which allows a unique perspective in seeing the imbalance in others. I must confess that this insight often has a blind spot directly over oneself. However, when occupying this fulcrum of balance, we can see that complete healing requires that the doctor must perform multiple roles. There is a continuum from doctor as scientist to counselor then to healer in which one must inhabit all aspects at the same time.

Somewhere along the development path of medicine and dentistry, there was a replacement of traditional healing with the concepts of infection, immunity, and bacteriology. The rapid advances in scientific medicine at the end of the nineteenth century, and well into modern times, have sufficiently supplanted the role of traditional medicine derived from centuries of observation along with trial and error. We still adhere to many of the criteria of infection established in the late 1800s by Robert Koch, as stipulated in Koch's Postulates (the four basic criteria to establish an infective agent). Due to the widespread practice of traditional medicines, the nascent scientific community at the time struggled to advance their ideas initially. In fighting the power of belief in traditional medicines, scientists of the time fought vociferously against many long-held traditions. This led to the positioning of science as the savior and vanguard of a new generation versus traditional medicine as a vestige of superstition and myth. Those armed with the scientific method eagerly sought to attack, disprove, and discredit the centuries of accumulated "old wives' tales." As a result, our popular society still has difficulty accepting the idea of a balance point being a destination. While many medications are ineffective at low levels and become poisonous at high amounts, the "therapeutic effect" balance point of medicines is the "porridge that's just right."

Nearly 150 years into this triumph of science over tradition, we are now beginning to look at what was inadvertently discarded with the discreditation of traditional methods of healing. Rather than the vanquishing of a traditional medicine demon, perhaps there is still value to the collected wisdom of centuries past. Per our previous section, it is quite clear that we have not maximized the power of belief in a standardized way in modern medicine.

In addition, there is something inherently intuitive about balance equating to health. "Moderation in all things" is attributed to the Greek poet Hesiod in about 700 BCE. A vast number of healing traditions involve the rebalancing of vital energies, such as *qi* (Chinese), *prana* (Hindu), *ruah* (Hebrew), *pneuma* (Greek), or *ka* (Egyptian). This idea of a vital essence that gives life to our physical bodies exist in cultures in the Middle East, Africa, Asia, islands of Oceania, Native Americas, Amazonian jungles, and Europe.

Many of these healing modalities further divided the vital essences into physical elements that roughly correspond to a rudimentary periodic table. Ayurvedic medicine, developed in India, spoke of balancing the *doshas*, the three vital energies that give life to our physical bodies. In ancient Greece and Rome, there was the idea of the balancing of *humors* within the body to attain health (some scholars believe that the idea of humors has their origin in Egypt or Mesopotamia). Chinese medicinal texts speak often of balancing the *yin* and *yang*, corresponding to the dark and light within us. This was recognition that all manner of things can be had in excess or deficit. In balance, we teeter upon the edge, demonstrating the fragility of life and the narrow set of physical parameters under which we are able to exist.

In my formative years, my grandmother occasionally relented and permitted a pestering impatient child to accompany her to the local traditional Chinese pharmacy. There I would marvel at the walls of drawers filled with meticulously collected and carefully dried medicinal plants, fungi, animal parts, and the errant cicada molting. The pungent aroma of the combinations of medicinal ingredients was sufficient to cement the experience in my long-term memory. Over time, it was explained to me that each medicine not only has an herbal value, it also has a nature represented by the shade and darkness (*yin*), or the light and heat (*yang*).

Under Traditional Chinese Medicine, the body has a normal flow of *qi* (pronounced "chee," roughly translated as "breath of life") that courses through the arteries and veins as a river. Imbalances induced by the environment or behavior of the patient would impede the natural flow of this vital essence. The medicinal mixture was to be determined by a doctor of Chinese Medicine, who tailored the ingredients to rebalance the *yin* and *yang*, thus clearing various blockages that caused obstructions. Naturally, this doctor would perform attentive observations on the tinge of one's facial complexion as well as careful examination of the pulse and heart rhythms. Remarkably, this practice was brought over to the United States by enterprising immigrants who continue to practice their healing arts with the love and compassion normally reserved for their own families.

We are no strangers to the idea of balance in order to achieve a state of health, yet its common practice seems elusive. It is a fair question whether the ubiquitous marketing campaigns for various industries and lobbies have been overly effective in countering our ultimate goal of equilibrium. To the world outside the United States, there is an incredulity to the belief that bigger is always better. Only in our country of plenty do we develop the idea that if more is better, then an overwhelming excess is surely the best. Alas, scores of children have attempted to prove this very theory with cookies, candy, and other assorted treats. Much to their dismay, there may be something to this idea of balance after all.

CHAPTER 14

The Root Necessities

Imbalance permeates our society as it exists in the western world. Entire lives are devoted to the extremes of the spectrum within many disciplines as we celebrate or ridicule the best and the worst of anything. Western society has abundant positives to offer, yet there are few examples of sustainable balance guiding us in our individual journeys through independence, freedom, and choice. While the Amazonian tribal communities learn from birth the value of balance in nature that sustains their water and food sources, our society of plentifulness cradles our youth in bubbles of security and protection. Even the daily trek to draw water from the river or spring presented the opportunity to emphasize the need to avoid soiling the sources. The indigenous communities require balance due to the thin edge upon which they survive.

In contrast, the abundance in many western societies removes the regular reminder of the delicate nature of our existence. Lacking from western childhoods are the many constant social cues that impress upon us the fine line upon which we exist in relative harmony with nature and her plants and animals. We seek to shape the world to do our bidding, limited only by the size of our bank accounts. Only with life experience do we look back and begin to moderate our youthful viewpoints. It is this milieu from which our patients emerge in various states of imbalance.

Regardless of spiritual upbringing, a similar set of concepts recur on the goals of various spiritual teachings. Chief among these life goals and most basic needs, we find peace, love, joy, and purpose. In order to understand the true nature of balance, a deeper understanding of these concepts is necessary. Many of our basic needs in life stem from these four basic principles. Once again, the goal is not to indulge in a comparative spiritual discourse but to build the structure from which we can extend our ability to empathize and rebalance elements within the lives of our patients and ourselves.

Peace extends to our need to have the space outside of conflict to grow and nurture ourselves and those we love. When we imagine inadequate peace, many of us have images of war-torn regions of our world with tired, dirty, injured or maimed, or even dead combatants lying in fields pockmarked with mortar explosions. Consider the idea that all-out fighting wars can essentially prevent us from attaining any of the basic concepts of peace, love, joy, and purpose. Peace itself is a prerequisite and foundational piece for any of the principles to survive and thrive. It is not to say that we cannot have love, joy, and purpose in a time of war, but the natural growth of these concepts is constantly disrupted and thus stunted over time. Of course, an actual war is a dramatic example worthy of many movie plots, but the idea of inadequate peace also can be seen in times of familial strife. For example, from a child's point of view, parents that constantly fight and argue severely disrupt the peace of the home. It affects not only the idea of the home as a safe place but also impacts the child's sense of identity and self-esteem. The regular overload of trauma can deeply scar a developing mind to the point of coloring and affecting all future decisions and choices.

Love is the need to express affection and deep acceptance for and from another single person or family group. To love and be loved is the most important part of feeling accepted and validated as a person worthy of love. There are many types of love that our literary tradition delves into extensively. We see romantic love, platonic love, love between siblings, love between family members, love between friends, love of animals, and so on... In many cases within our society, romantic love is held up as a shining beacon that trumps all other goals. However, we would be remiss in leaving out the role of the many other types of love that enrich our lives. Indeed, the need to feel affection and contact is a trait not exclusive to humans. We can also genuinely feel the love from animals and other sentient beings that share our world.

As healthcare professionals, we will rarely delve into the deeper aspects of love when dealing with patients. However, through our care, we show the capacity for such a love. Many of us show our love for people in the effort that we display toward helping our patients, or in the passion in our work, and this is essential to establishing the common human connection and contact. We "hold" our patients metaphorically and sometimes physically through our caring for their overall well-being. Great pains must be taken to communicate that we choose to serve others to show love for people and the world around us. There is such a deficit of this quality in our collective upbringing that it has become a worldwide need. As such, it is the most likely universal point of contact.

Joy refers to the spark of happiness that occurs while engaging in any chosen experience. The delight in engaging chosen activities is a clear indicator of joy. In children of all ages, it is simply the pleasure of choosing something that fulfills everything that we need at the moment. It can be attained by many methods, including the attainment of a goal or dream, the embrace of anything that reminds us of a beloved activity or person, or even the appreciation of being somewhere resolutely beautiful. Joy is the reward that we receive for making a good choice or being in the right place at the right time. It can involve getting a result that far exceeds our expectations. It is also reveling in the amazement of realizing that we are connected by a grander scheme than what we had previously known. We see it in the faces of children when they discover something new. It is all these things and more as it relates to pure happiness.

Purpose is the need to not only be necessary, but to be integral to a part of something greater than just ourselves. Imagine a group of philosophers in togas gathering to discuss the meaning of life. These existential questions can be seen as purely academic but on a practical level, it is essential to state our immediate goals yet have a larger umbrella of a mission statement or stated purpose to our lives. It is the ultimate validation of our necessity in the world around us. In the grand scheme, it gives us the reason for our existence, yet it can be as small as doing a job for a minute. Purpose guides us in our daily endeavors. In an instance of deficiency, we may feel frustration at not having our talents utilized efficiently or feeling aimless without a goal. People or groups without a purpose generally engage in haphazard activity without the order and structure necessary to affect a specific goal. Conversely, when purpose is in excess over long term, we experience a progressive overstimulation and feeling of too much weight on your shoulders. This in turn can lead to frustration, burnout, and long-term scarring that reaches into the subconscious mind. Of course, there is much variation in where the balance resides in each element.

CHAPTER 15

The Nature *of* Coping Mechanisms

Considering the case of Claire from Chapter 10, it is apparent that we all have different capacities to deal with our problems. Usually, the number of tasks on our plate is directly proportional to the amount of stress in our lives. While stress in mild to moderate amounts is a basic mechanism to initial adaptation, there is again a threshold after which we see physical and mental degradation.

From our discussion of memory decay and its role as a coping mechanism, we are able to witness some of the methods by which our bodies and minds naturally attempt to fix their own problems. There is a self-regulatory character that seems to stem from our survival instinct which extends from physical healing of a wound to the psyche coping with cumulative damage. We can see some evidence of this in mice studies with the increasing self-administration of dopamine stimulants (ethanol, in this particular study) as well as corticosteroids in the presence of increasing stress.[63] This self-medication is a behavioral adaptation to decrease the severity of the stress insult by activating the reward pathways. Modifications of these types incorporate many levels of behavioral change.

There appear to be levels to the coping mechanisms. As we take a deeper look at the processes involved in coping, it becomes useful to look at pain models. When dealing with pain, there is the initial mechanism of emotional adaptation. People experiencing mild pain will tell themselves that it is bearable, and they can handle it without changing their normal behavior. There is a mental rationalization of the painful experience that convinces a person that being able to withstand the pain is an indicator for their toughness and worthiness. They may even equate the pain with another beneficial process, as in a weight training scenario (No pain, no gain!).

Upon experiencing moderate pain, the emotional state may seek to increase its coping mechanisms. Physical activation of the body's natural stress relief with the glucocorticoid system is upregulated. At the limits of emotional coping, the tolerance for the pain begins to take a turn, and the subject's mood changes for the worse. The beginnings of behavioral modifications to commence self-medication with chemicals and medications are not uncommon at this point. Consider the popularity of painkillers among members of any local gym or sporting venue.

Somewhere in the vicinity of moderate pain, there is a threshold after which emotional coping is wholly inadequate. When this threshold is surpassed, any further progression of the pain is perceived as advanced, and the coping mechanism switches to a physical nature. If the pain can be avoided physically, the subject will adjust their behavior to keep a physical distance away from any related stimulus that will cause the pain. The previous reference to a spider bite phobia fits into this situation perfectly in that the mind is programmed to avoid any similar exposure to spiders. In the case that physical avoidance is not possible, mental dissociation will arise as an option.[64]

Coping mechanisms are effective up to a threshold, after which we can detect deleterious effects on the brain. There is a whole spectrum of ways that the body utilizes to cope with the increasing severity of the stress or insult. In the event the stress or insult greatly exceeds the body's ability to cope, we begin to see a breakdown of the normal processes of everyday memory, learning, interpersonal relations, and socialization. Changes in the DNA associated with extreme stress have been documented[65], and classified as *epigenetic changes* (environment induced changes to the genome).[66] Studies in animal models as well as in humans are very clear in the aftereffects of overwhelming stresses, with Post- Traumatic Stress Disorder (PTSD) symptoms, including but not limited to cue-induced fear behavior, depression, rage, anxiety, and insomnia.[67] Only recently has this more comprehensive idea of PTSD been able to allow a new approach to treatment.

When we look at evidence linking extreme psychological trauma to stress then to actual detectable damage in the brain, it begins to dawn on us that the levels of brain injury exist as a continuum. This continuum begins where our coping abilities are exhausted and ends with clear disruption of normal cognitive, behavioral, and memory capacities. On the other end of the severity spectrum, we have physical injury to the brain due to repeated impact. Interest in this area has spiked within the recent timeframe specifically due to chronic traumatic encephalopathy (CTE) in concussion cases related to athletes. In those cases, repeated physical brain trauma leads to a detectable increase in damage indicators (proteinopathy) within the brain when compared with healthy brain tissue.[68]

While the CTE cases appear to be extremes on our spectrum of brain damage, there are usually much more mild conditions with which we may come into contact. Provided we are not recognizing the severity of the damage, and thus not initiating treatment, these damages can accumulate quickly. If we assess the trauma threshold of a patient, we can then individualize our potential treatment plans to specifically reprioritize pain control and sedation in those susceptible low-threshold patients.

Many chronic issues involving the psyche are misguided self-treatment of imbalances aimed at the symptoms. In the case of trauma, our coping mechanisms for the initial trauma allowed us to survive the incident, but the continued activation of that coping mechanism outside the situation where it was necessary leads to a dysfunction. This unregulated repetition multiplied over numerous traumas can complicate any treatment significantly. The symptom is treated, but the root imbalance is not addressed. To complicate matters, there is the entire branch of "epigenetics," which describes how the human genome allows for different genes to be activated based on the environmental factors faced. The classic debate between nature versus nurture (DNA vs. environment) has been answered by an emphatic yes to both.

Aside from the physical injuries to the brain, psychological stresses are a major stimulus that elicits a reaction from the coping mechanisms. The mind automatically reacts in a type of self-treatment in an attempt to balance or manage the daily stresses and perceived attacks to which people are subject to in daily interactions. For example, an obnoxious patient begins to annoy the receptionist in your office. Her initial reaction is to feel the irritation that automatically leads her to avoid the man or to tell him to cut out the noxious behavior. Unmanaged reactions to an initial insult will often be self-preserving by nature but will be inadequate in the face of repeated damage. Should the obnoxious patient continue his assault on the receptionist over time, inaction on the part of management creates a toxic work environment. Psychologists are only now studying the effects of accumulated "microaggressions" experienced in the daily lives of racial minority groups.[69] Active management of the coping response must be present for us to have the necessary ingredients for proper healing.

One prime example of the intertwined nature of coping and addiction was studied extensively by Harvey Milkman, a psychology professor who examined coping mechanisms in teenagers in Colorado.[70] In his doctoral dissertation, he studied the preferences in teenagers for heroin (an opiate which depresses the senses and gives a numbing effect) versus amphetamines (which stimulates and excites one to confront their stresses).[71] He found that the drug preference was significantly dependent on the type of personality of the teen. The heroin abuser uses the sedative effect for repression and withdrawal, while the amphetamine addict stimulates themselves to "maintain a posture of active confrontation with the environment." These self-treatments appeared to temporarily aid in the reduction of anxiety borne from the primal need for self-preservation.

We now know that a combination of both genetics and neurobiology separate these two basic types of personalities: the externalizing pathway and the internalizing pathway. The externalizing pathway is characterized by the need for impulse and risk with a greater likelihood of being sensation and reward-seeking. Examples of this pathway may include "persistent disobedience, stealing, aggression, vandalism, gang fighting, and homicide."[72] In other words, there is an underlying "inability to inhibit socially undesirable or restricted actions."[73] The internalizing pathway tends more toward introversion and wires the person to cope with negative emotions like fear and anger. Individuals tending toward this pathway often struggle with depression, social dissociation, and general anxiety.

Milkman's ideas were put to the test in 1992 when he won a grant to start Project Self-Discovery, which was aimed at developing reducing the rate of teenage drug addiction and crime.[74] The project examined the coping mechanisms of the teenagers and replaced their drugs of choice with activities that produced the natural highs that addressed their particular neurological needs. The enrolled teenagers were given a choice of activities that would alter their brain chemistry to give them the effect of either stimulating a rush or dealing with anxiety. Instructors were brought in for a range of activities including dance, music, martial arts, carpentry, and anything the teens wanted to learn.

In the previous year, Milkman had piqued the interest of a residential drug treatment center in the city of Tindar, Iceland. In response to some of the highest rates of youth drinking in Europe, the Icelandic government was looking for solutions. In 1992, 1995, and 1997, they gave a questionnaire to every 14-, 15-, and 16-year-old in their school system to inquire on their experience and involvement with drugs, alcohol, cigarettes, preferred activities, and time spent with family. Alarmingly, the results showed that teenage alcohol abuse was rampant in the country, with nearly 42% admitting to being drunk at least once in the past month. 23% identified as daily smokers, and 17% registered cannabis usage.

Further analysis of the data from the surveys also showed drastic differences between the teens that delved into smoking, drugs, and alcohol, and those that remained sober. Apparently, organized sports, time spent with parents, avoiding being outdoors in the late evenings, and feeling cared about at school were strongly associated with protecting the teens who abstained from the addictive habits.

Using this data and the recommendations of researchers including Milkman, the Icelandic government formulated a plan called Youth in Iceland. They proceeded to implement their recommendations in every school to address all their findings and encourage the positive activities that allowed the teens to avoid the worst habits. The laws were changed to ban tobacco and alcohol advertisements, and limited tobacco purchases to 18 years and over, and alcohol to 20 years and over. Curfews were enacted for 13- to 16-year-olds to 10 p.m. in the winter and midnight in the summer. State funding was increased to teach the range of activities that were effective in helping the teens cope.

So spectacular was their success that nearly every negative metric decreased and all the positive indicators such as time spent with parents and time spent in organized sports nearly doubled within five years.

The Icelandic model shows that a rebalancing of an entire society to healthier activities is possible. They were able to implement the steps of assessment, analysis, and feeding the deficiencies with a comprehensive "whole-of-government" approach. While this is not practical nor possible in many places, it shows that when you feed a person or a group what they need, many of their dysfunctions resolve. Whether we emphasize stimulation or anxiety relief, we are introducing better ways to cope with stress and anxiety. Rather than working against the natural tendencies dictated by both genetics and the environment, we can go with the grain of human psychology, and our patients will begin to thrive. Much like in caring for an infant, when we fulfill a need, they continue to grow normally. When we are unaware of or ignore a vital need, the infant can only cry or act up.

CHAPTER 16

The Art *of* Achieving Balance

The main point of achieving balance is to occupy the space from which you have an unparalleled perspective of the range of internal and external influences that divert people away from their stated priorities. Many of the external influences come from social interactions in our lives along with the selective activation of memories. In past generations, it has been print and television advertising that swayed public opinion on ideas of fashion, style, propriety, and even morality. Increasingly, social networking programs have been wreaking havoc on the natural tendencies of populations and deftly utilizing the neurological reward systems to further their profit line. One significant challenge in our jobs is that a capitalistic system such as ours favors extremes in behavior. These extremes are often counter to our ideas of balance. In essence, we are fighting a mass marketing machine that constantly tells our patients that they are not enough, too fat, or too ugly to be happy unless they take this pill, injection, or surgery to fix their problem. Our society may not see this as a major problem at this point, yet once separated from the media and marketing, thousands of American children in wilderness camps return to a different baseline of mental health. On my visits to indigenous communities across the world, the absence of the marketing within their social spheres draws a drastic contrast to Western idea of "normal."

On the smaller scale, it is not uncommon for patients to ask us our opinions on their health decisions. Our ability to cut through the confusion and chaos of our patient's lives and sort through their priorities will further reinforce their trust in our relationship, thus strengthening our capacity to help them.

With the aforementioned concepts, we must now consider the age-old idea of balance. Balance can refer to a state of stable health, of course, but it also extends to the criteria of peace, love, joy, and purpose, as well as other more complex needs that determine our idea of fulfillment. And before we can really begin to pursue balance for our patients, we must achieve it ourselves.

While Western society has a penchant for shifting the external view, Eastern cultures delve deeply into the internal aspect. As a matter of approach, both sample a wide breadth of the human experience. Combined together, they have the capacity to unite disparate opinions and defuse the enmity between deeply entrenched antagonists. It is therefore no mystery that we carry our views with us, wearing them boldly on our sleeves. This in turn affects those around us and influences the ability of others to hear our suggestions and receive our communications to them. In order to have our medical advice accepted and followed, it helps to look the part of a compassionate and wise caretaker. For us to gain access to the most receptive audiences, there is a need to balance our own internal and external routines and rhythms. If we do not attain a reasonable balance within ourselves, we will lack the requisite reference point from which to assess and diagnose anyone else. Below is my personal three-stage process that I have found helpful for attaining and sustaining internal balance for both patient and doctor.

Recover:

Recognize how you feel at the moment. This is not to begin a philosophical meditation accompanied by soft contemplative music and yoga pants. Instead, acknowledgment that your feelings are a communication from your subconscious mind will allow you to assess the kinds of sensory details collected. Check in with your subconscious to determine if there are any lingering issues that you have not yet processed thoroughly. Be mindful of where you stand at this particular moment physically, where you stand in your goals, life, and relationships, and the resulting stance you have taken to face the world around. Take note of your energy levels and how well rested you are. When we are rested, we generally tend to be in a more positive mood.

The mood is an excellent indicator of how tired we may feel. Often, we disregard our feelings and continue to push ourselves to fulfill expectations and goals. Fatigue can lead us into not only a foul state of mind but also to poor decision-making, enabling certain negative reactions to things that we otherwise handle easily. This fatigue decreases our performance in many aspects and our threshold for overload decreases and overall awareness suffers. In addition, our speed and ability to process subtle body language and visualize unhealthy patterns within our patients becomes impaired.

Take inventory of the burdens that you carry every day and consider the unspoken expectations that you bring. There are also daily traumas in our life that we brush aside. Have you come to terms with these traumas, or are they still lingering? For example, I have colleagues whose routine discussions with their parents present such a power struggle and negative imaging that they are often exhausted from being in their presence. Their awareness of everything else immediately afterward is overwhelmed by the traumatic experience. Ensure adequate rest and recover from the fatigue that impairs our awareness skills.

Recall and Review:

Recall and review the negative feelings that are underlying our daily lives such as anger, annoyance, fear of failing, missing deadlines, and under-performing goals. Count the number of baseline burdens that are present even as you are sitting in your office. How much is the overhead cost every day to keep an office open; how busy is our work schedule; are there any deadlines; are there any conflicts between your employees? Questions of these types should not add to your stresses, as whatever the status, it has already happened. This is the baseline that we start with on a daily basis.

Reset:

When we are able to assess the items and burdens we subconsciously carry with us everywhere, we can start to shift the negative energy into a positive direction. Break down your burdens to one thing at a time and give them a priority. We all vary as far as our multitasking abilities. I always remember a scene in a Western movie where the protagonist cowboy shoots six or eight gunslingers in a bar all at once—or so it seemed. Upon recounting the episode, he explained that careful observation allowed him to prioritize the opponents by their likelihood of shooting first. Then he calmly progressed down his target selection going in the order of his priority list. Of course, he did it in such a smooth manner that it appeared to bystanders as if he had shot them all at once.

Only allow one issue (or any number you feel comfortable with) to come through the door at any specific moment in time. Prioritize our burdens and place them in a single file line. This sequencing is not to suggest that you cannot multitask but is for the purpose of resetting your subconscious mind. Breathe deliberately and slowly to establish a rhythm. As we count the items passing through our doorway, consider what it looks and feels like to have each item succeed brilliantly beyond your expectations. Feel the happiness and relief of meeting and surpassing your goals. Engage the feeling of impending celebration in response to your successes. When we convert the negative feelings into positive action, we will mobilize and enable our full capabilities to engage something that our subconscious tells us is important. Listening to our subconscious allows us to check in with ourselves to see if there is anything that we missed and might skew our judgment while assessing patients. We have a way of confusing and projecting our own feelings into the problems of others that is not only confusing to a bystander but will prevent us from using all our senses in the practice of medicine, dentistry, and healing in general. Recognize that the mere act of asking these questions commences the reset of your subconscious mind for the moment and centers your observational energies to achieve the hyperawareness necessary for keen insight.

Ultimately, the goal of reestablishing objectivity is to detach oneself from your personal perspective and adopt the bird's eye overview of your own life. By reviewing all the underlying thoughts that dominate our busy lives, we can begin to simplify our intentions. If we can effectively recognize and minimize our internal biases and prejudices, we may come to view events and actions as they exist individually, rather than emotionally linked to any patterns. This clarity of view not only allows improvements in awareness internally but makes us externally more approachable by others. To paraphrase the eminent American Buddhist scholar, Ven. Bhikkhu Bodhi, the point of internal balance for meditation is attaining the point of awareness where we have reached a state of full wakefulness, unaccompanied by the chatter of conscious thinking.[75]

With this grounding, we can return to our driving purpose for our patients. We seek to achieve balance and thus a healthy sustainable outcome by feeding the deficiencies that we can perceive in them, then observing for the desired outcome. Consider the idea of an old-fashioned scale with a balance point in the center and a basket tied to both ends. In order to achieve balance, we can either make the heavier side lighter, or the lighter side heavier. We can also change the point of fulcrum. As such, this relates to the idea of damage inhabiting one side of the scale, and healing on the opposite side. Whenever the scales are balanced, we have a sustained state of no change. However, the damage side can be adversely affected by harmful exposure to disease-causing elements, wear and tear, incompletely healed injuries, inadequate nutrition, and aging. In the case of periodontal disease, there are proven genetic deficiencies that make certain patients break down faster than others.[76] The host response is also a condition where the immune system's normal defense mechanisms are turned into a destructive element.

The healing side of the scale is inhabited by the body's natural ability to heal, including adequate nutrition (good diet), adequate healing time, active reduction of known damaging substances (bacterial, viral, and chemical), and more recently biological and chemical mediators for healing, such as growth factors, supportive proteins, and biostimulation radiation. Due to aging being a constant for our physical bodies, the equation tilts toward the side of damage more often than stasis or healing. It is a constantly changing equation for which we must counteract the effects of aging by constantly improving on the healing side to even maintain a stasis situation. This idea applies to many but certainly not all chronic diseases, as the multifactorial aspects confound even the most ardent scientists.

When we are dealing with a chronic disease, there is a general trend of minor imbalance in the scale towards the side of damage exceeding that of healing. In other words, the scale tends to tip more toward damage than healing. Consider also that this may not necessarily be a steady constant breakdown. There are numerous instances in medicine and dentistry (e.g. diabetes, periodontitis) where most damage is incurred in episodes between long periods of relative stability. In major imbalances, rapid decline of the host patient is expected due to excessive damage overwhelming the healing response. Debilitating diseases often follow this pattern of downward spiraling culminating in the ultimate success of the damage. The element of time and the point at which we are seeing the patient is critical to our assessment. The increments of time during which we are involved in the care of the patient may change our perception of the rate of breakdown.

Some of the most common feelings faced by patients are impatience and frustration. From the standpoint of understanding the communication and responding appropriately, both frustration and impatience stem from the expectation of being further along in progress than where they find themselves. Both feelings can be remedied by either improving the outcome time (which isn't always possible) or changing the expectation of the anticipated treatment time.

In order to achieve balance of more complex needs for our patients, we must first recognize the areas in which they are in excess or in deficiency. These are not necessarily opposing forces that are at odds with one another, although that is possible. For example, a person may be experiencing a long period of peace which triggers yearnings for excitement and adventure. It may also trigger a wanderlust for travel and personal growth. This is a natural response by the subconscious to self-regulate by driving the desire for something that is needed emotionally. Rebalancing can be as subtle as a suggestion for our patients to listen to their subconscious needs. In this way, we merely serve as a guide that gives them permission to pursue what their subconscious is already telling them.

Another example of an imbalance can be seen in someone who has an excess of purpose. In our modern world, we have a system of commerce that is dependent on producing and having more. This inevitably leads to a work life that is often hectic and overbooked with goals, deadlines, and expectations. Many unrealized ideas continue to nag at us as something that remains necessary for our perceived success. This is purpose that we place on ourselves, as well as placed on us by employers, managers, and companies. We place the pressure on ourselves to be the link between utter failure and brilliant success. Of course, we can be overwhelmed with purpose in our lives. Fortunately, purpose will often have a timeline, after which the pressure to perform reduces. In these cases, our method to rebalance may be as simple as telling our patients to "take it easy" after the next project is done. We may bring their attention to the effects of stress on their body, teeth, etc. An important aspect is also to recognize that this patient may be addicted to overwhelming purpose because it also serves a need in their subconscious mind. They may be responding to a prior experience of inadequate purpose or purpose hinging on self-worth.

We must ensure that when feeding the deficiency we do not accidently feed an addiction (defined as a negative cycle of coping). These addictions tend to come from an external source and are often deleterious to overall well-being. For example, a person who is lonely will seek friends on social media. It is well known that social media platforms employ a framework for advertisement to a captive audience.[77] The programing of the software purposefully seeks to present periodic exposure to things or events that you may find enjoyable or reinforce what you already believe. In ensuring regular exposure, there is a measured neurotransmitter release in the brain (dopamine) that is associated with feeling good. By controlling the amount of dopamine your brain releases over time, the desired result is to affect a longer duration of exposure to advertisements on their platform.

The increase in use of social media, while giving the outward appearance of immense popularity, may decrease the actual meaningful human relationships formed. This in turn leads the individual to seek more social media friends, and likely withdraw from the flesh-and-blood type. In many ways, this mimics the response of the human body to addictive drugs. Consider the manipulation of a basic human response (loneliness) gives the appearance of having many friends on social media. This fills a perceived need with a mismatched solution without true tangible value.

With these companies actively exploiting the dopamine reward system to increase their addictive qualities, it is strikingly similar to the strategies employed by the tobacco companies to expand their market share in the 1950s through the 1990s.

If we can project the eventual outcome of no intervention, then we can start to see the degree of imbalance in the patient. Sometimes staying the course is an effective option, especially when time will automatically resolve an issue. However, doing nothing in the face of a progressively worsening condition will have serious negative consequences. Looking at the current course, can you anticipate where that patient will stand given a specific period of time?

Ethically, the course of treatment should ultimately be determined by the patient. As medical practitioners, we have the responsibility to give patients options, make recommendations, and lay out our process in coming to our conclusions. This allows the patient to take responsibility for their own path in treatment. In this manner, patients tend to remain more engaged, as they are deeply invested in the decision-making process. It also allows room to deflect any later blame should a patient change their mind.

If there is a commonality between our own imbalances and that of our patients (perhaps a shared history of addiction), it gives us an entry point into the conversation with our patients. Common experiences resonate with people and leads to a feeling of connection and establishes a point of contact. This contact is significant when both healer and patient can relate to each other on even ground. There is no outside judgment involved, as the perceived parity between both the patient and healthcare practitioner removes any threatening atmosphere. Without the power disparity, a doorway opens for the patient to ask the question "How did you get through it?" If the healthcare practitioner does not establish contact, any comments may be perceived by patient as an attack or judgement from an external source. Another point of contact must be quickly established in order to continue this communication. Should a conversation veer into this direction, intervening and resetting the stage will be necessary to reestablish the connection. Reaching back to common experiences from a close relative or friend emphasizes the feeling of caring. This empathy is a necessity, and any other points where they can relate to each other will be helpful in this regard. For example, a doctor who practices martial arts can relate his personal experience of trying to train despite having a broken rib to a patient who has just suffered a frustrating sports injury.

The power to rebalance yourself allows you to stay in the zone where you can observe the imbalances in others. We do not inherently know the feeling of this point of balance as our coping mechanisms allow us to get accustomed to many situations including unbalanced ones. If we can find this balance point, however, and remember this as the baseline for health, we can return to this point again. This baseline is important as a reference point both for us and for relating to a patient with a similar problem. When we present our perspective from this viewpoint to a patient as the baseline, any deviation that we bring up can then be more accepted by the patient so long as they do not feel that the criticism is with the intent to attack. The contact, in this case, is ensuring that the patient knows your intent is benign and aimed at enabling their self-improvement. The presence of this contact is the critical defining factor between your comments being perceived as constructive criticism, or a destructive judgment.

As we come to incrementally understand the psychological patterns at play in how we face medicine, healthcare, and illness, we can start to formulate an action plan and flow chart for navigating the complex framework of the human mind.

In Figure 1., we take all the signs and symptoms and categorize them into three main types: 1) Physical manifestation only (black), 2) Physical manifestation with behavioral imbalances (white), and 3) Root behavioral causes (gray). The black boxes represent injuries and diseases where we can trace a definitive cause. This may be a physical injury like a broken leg due to falling out of a tree, or an infection of known bacterial or viral cause. For these self-limiting situations, direct treatment of the injury or disease will suffice.

The white boxes initially present as a physical injury except for the presence of a detectable behavioral imbalance or a repeated pattern. An appropriate example is the condition of bulimia. Patients suffering from this type of eating disorder will present with massive dental erosion and decay on an otherwise young and seemingly healthy person. Upon seeing these patients, we need to treat the immediate damage as well as address the underlying behavioral issues that lead to perpetuation of the vomiting cycles. Another classic example is poor diabetic control where poor management of blood sugar is due to diet and exercise imbalances. In addition to stabilizing the current blood sugar imbalance, there is a need to determine the behavioral support necessary to achieve regularly successful diabetes management.

The gray boxes represent the purely behavioral issues that may not have an immediately treatable physical problem. Examples include mood, impulse-control, anxiety, stress-related disorders, and substance-related disorders. The initial line of questioning will be aimed at identifying the key characteristics of the behavior and determining how it may subconsciously be serving an unspoken need. Bringing awareness to and reconciling the discrepancies between the conscious mind and the subconscious needs will allow the decoupling and disempowerment of the behavior. Are there alternatives to filling the needs that do not involve the disadvantages or consequences of the unwanted behavior?

FIGURE 1. FACILITATING HEALING THROUGH BALANCE

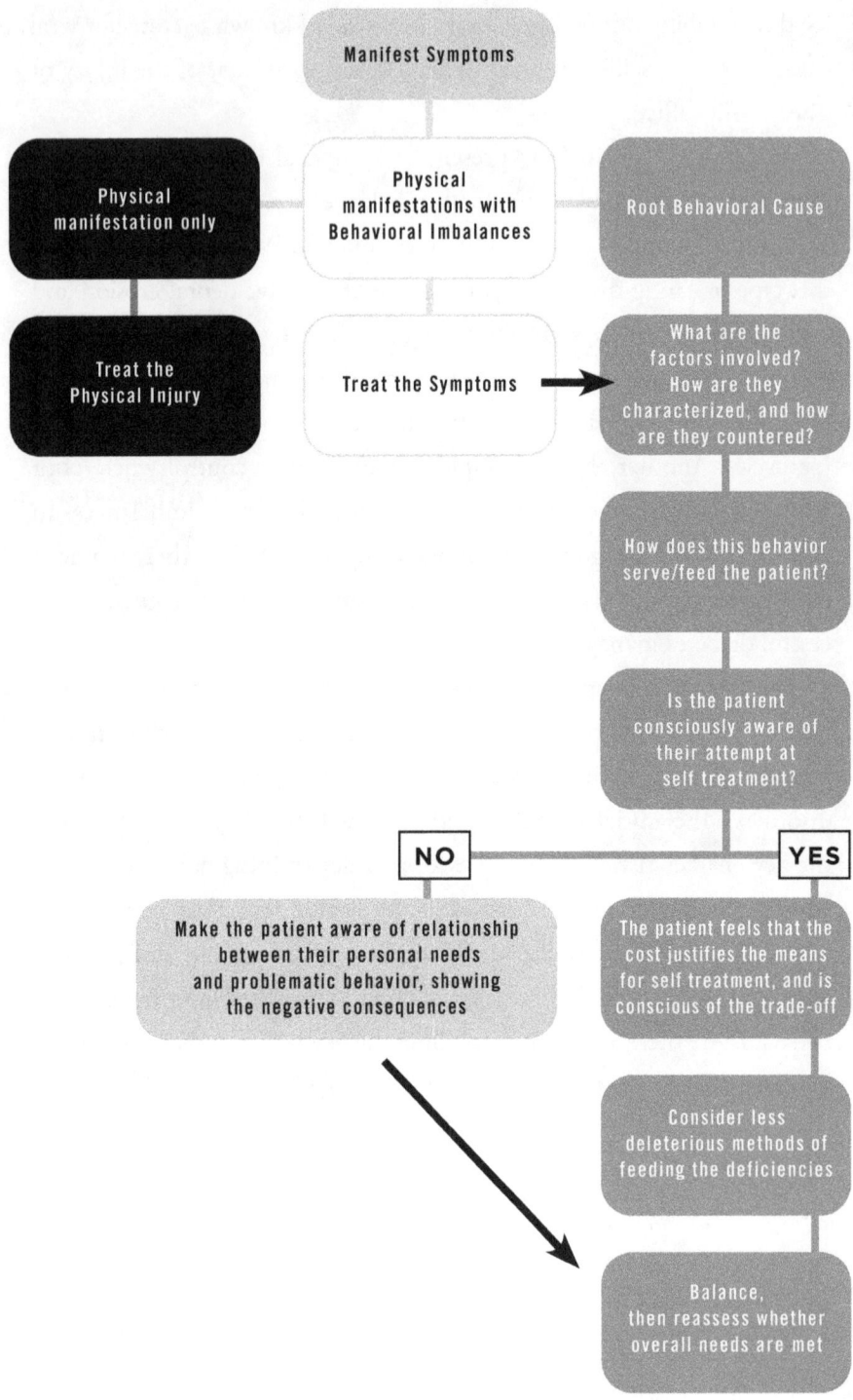

Manifest Symptoms

Physical manifestation only

Physical manifestations with Behavioral Imbalances

Root Behavioral Cause

Treat the Physical Injury

Treat the Symptoms

What are the factors involved? How are they characterized, and how are they countered?

How does this behavior serve/feed the patient?

Is the patient consciously aware of their attempt at self treatment?

NO

YES

Make the patient aware of relationship between their personal needs and problematic behavior, showing the negative consequences

The patient feels that the cost justifies the means for self treatment, and is conscious of the trade-off

Consider less deleterious methods of feeding the deficiencies

Balance, then reassess whether overall needs are met

CHAPTER 17

Addictive Behavior

During the course of our practice, we come across many patients who have strong personalities who enjoy dictating the method and speed of treatment. Some even manage to make excellent choices and match our internal professional opinions. The likelihood of success is high when we have motivated patients that know exactly what they want. These convictions may be deeply held beliefs that are reinforced by numerous positive outcomes and may be deeply learned lessons that serve as guiding philosophies over a lifetime. Dealing with individuals with strong beliefs or convictions is quite manageable as their parameters are already drawn, and they are usually not shy in informing you of their boundaries.

The more difficult question is how do you discern a strong personality with that of a pathological condition? That line between the healthy and the addicted is drawn at the point of a person knowingly suffering damage to themselves in order to achieve a goal. If that goal is ultimately positive, our society forgives the addictive behavior, and the deleterious effects become a badge of strength and willingness to sacrifice. We define addictions as behavior that is repeated despite being fully aware of its negative consequences. It is no surprise that addiction dominates our society as we glorify the vast capacity to suffer among the military, mainstream sports, endurance athletes, and even local gyms. From this cross section of our communities come the drug-seeking patients that create so many problems for the Drug Enforcement Agency.

The other shoe drops when overall negative effects begin to arise. Many people teeter on this edge between the positive effects of heavy exercise and the enduring physical pain of injury. The normalization of anti-inflammatory medications and painkillers has even hollowed out some of our societies' most celebrated heroes. With this in mind, their recovery is also based on achieving a balance that avoids the deleterious effects. In looking closer at the psychology and the neurology of the brain in these cases, we can demystify the disorder of addictions to reveal the underlying issues. As we look further into the biology of this condition, we will see that it is a dysfunction of the dopamine reward system that is normally a critical part of the learning mechanisms. Clearly, the normal functions have been hijacked to a progressive negative effect.

Our concept of addiction refers to any choice that we make repeatedly despite its negative effects on us and our relationships with others. This can include chemical dependence as the root causes are similar. Much like other learned experiences that bury themselves into our subconscious mind, addictions can be difficult when looking for the cause. In general, the main idea is that the addictive behavior serves a subconscious need for the patient. The underlying need is the true imbalance at the root of the problem. However, illicit drugs complicate the situation with the physical changes that deepen the cravings in addiction.

Within the brain, the biological basis for addictions and addictive behavior appears to be an over-reliance on the dopamine reward pathway. As discussed earlier, particular activities can elicit a consistent response within the regions of the brain involved with reward. Under normal circumstances, the dopamine reward system is activated in learning, memory, emotion, motivation, and pleasure. When drug addiction is involved, it overstimulates the brain's reward centers with dopamine and creates a euphoric effect colloquially known as a high. Researchers have found that certain drugs can lead to the multiplying of dopamine receptors, which initially increases the euphoria.[78] This appears to be a conditioning response to the flooding of dopamine much like the strengthening of a muscle that gets exercised. However, upon prolonged exposure, the receptors decrease in sensitivity, thus requiring more of the drug to elicit the same high intensity. Thus a person seeking the desired high will need to take increasing amounts of the drug just to create the same high as the first time. This destructive cycle is a slippery slope that leads to addiction and shows the power of the drug's hold. However, how much of the addiction is related to physiology, and how much of it involves psychology?

In a landmark study of Vietnam veterans returning from the war in 1971, Robins et al. surveyed 943 men and their experience with heroin and opium during and after their tours of duty.[79] He found that 45% of those surveyed noted experimentation with heroin or opium while on the front lines. Twenty percent of the soldiers reported addiction to opiates while in Vietnam, while only 11% tested positive for opiates upon their return. In following veterans addicted to opiates up to three years after their return, only 12% had relapsed. When we look at these numbers, there is more at play than just the physical addictive mechanisms. It appears that the heroin or opium served as a coping mechanism during combat, but the vast majority stopped their drug use upon returning to civilian life. Without the stress of war, being away from home in an unfamiliar environment, and what seemed like imminent death, nearly 90% of the returning soldiers no longer felt the need to dull the pain by self-medicating with opiates.

In examining the behavioral addictions, we are working with the same mechanisms, only to a slightly lesser degree. There are a myriad of things and behaviors to which we can become addicted. We have come to understand that anything that is enjoyable can become addictive. PET and fMRI imaging studies have confirmed that the same part of the brain responsible for drug addictions are also at play in other behavioral addictions.[80] In food addicts, the same areas within the brain associated with the reward centers in chemical addiction are activated. When there is stimulation on the lips, tongue, cheeks, and throat, the activated nerves in these areas stir up the physical and psychological memories of eating, and the subsequent flooding of dopamine into the pleasure centers. Eating is only one of many stimuli that your brain registers as a pleasurable experience. It is this common pathway to the reward and pleasure centers that may explain the number of people with multiple addictions, such as smoking and drinking, or gambling and sex.

To traditional healers, the idea of addictions is not limited to the realm of drug abuse. Addictive behavior is seen as an outward presentation of an internal imbalance. While much of the science is devoted to study of specific individual addictions, such as alcohol, food, gambling, and sex, there are many other behavioral addictions that are also in play. For example, some of the more common issues are obsessive-compulsive disorder (OCD), conflict, judgment, righteousness, control, power, use-fulness, powerlessness, or intelligence. Any of these can be issues in excess or deficiency. The need to feel the pleasure of the reward system creates a feedback loop that seems to alter the normal behavior of a person. This leads to the person continually seeking the situations that feed the perceived need, ignoring the deleterious effects to the rest of their lives. Quite a few of these are also ego-related and are attached to the idea of choices being or becoming your identity.

Addictive behavior can be rooted in the child development stage. When we look back at the mind and brain development, we can view the different types of traumas that can lead to later impairment. Typically, the greater the awareness of the child at the time of the trauma, the more impactful it becomes. Due to the extended period of development of the ego, many of the sources of mental imbalances are rooted in traumas to the idea of the child's developing self. These traumas may vary and can be as innocent as a critical comment of a judgmental adult on something that a child loves and to which he/she is deeply attached. One example is if a child loves to write, and their literary creation is criticized or dismissed as inadequate or unworthy. This wounding of the child is internalized and the criticism is relived over and over again until the only solution is that they are both inadequate and unworthy. A child in this situation may feel a subconscious lack of confidence whenever composing any written creation, or even avoid situations where they will be asked to write, as the long-ago criticism still stings.

Another example involves a child whose parents are extremely busy. The child finds early on that their only way of gaining attention for their basic needs would be by acting obnoxious and creating noise. This original wounding comes from neglect of the child during their time of need, and the solution for the child is to act out and become the "squeaky wheel." Often you will see that there is a subconscious-driven need to be the center of attention by annoying others. This initial wounding of the ego is reciprocated by the learned response of creating a scene and annoying everyone.

Much of the time, there is a strange sense of twisted logic to the conditions that our minds present to justify certain behavior that becomes learned and incorporated into everyday personalities. It is the logic of an incompletely developed mind that carries over into adulthood. You may see that many imbalances that are induced in childhood can later develop into addictions. Note that psychological addictions have a similar mechanism but differ slightly than chemical addictions to drugs. These psychological addictions are choices that we continue to make despite the negative effects.

When viewing addiction as a repeated choice that is made despite the negative side effects, our obvious question is "why?" Is it an intellectual equation where the perceived gain is seen as necessary while the negative effects are either inconsequential or manageable? Perhaps, but often the answer lies in the subconscious mind and its desire to feed a perceived need. The choices a person makes often reveals a fundamental aspect of their character that does not change easily. Repeated choices continually reinforce one's identity, and the other choices to the contrary will automatically be dismissed. These addictions over time can become part of our container, hence our identity.

Let us take conflict, for example. For those who revel in conflict, we may see them attempt to start conflicts within all their relationships whether business or personal. The idea of conflict is to gain an advantage by creating chaos. These are the situations when a person will create an argument for the sake of watching their opponents react to the attack. When breaking down and attacking opponents, the conflict-obsessed individual looks for opportunities to take advantage of when others are out of their element. It feeds the ego when the conflict-initiator holds their composure when everyone else is confused or on the defense. In the chaos, opportunities arise for the conflict-initiator to skip the order and decorum of civil discourse to take what they desired. This type of alpha personality individual tends to be very goal oriented and dominates most of their relationships.

Judgment is another of the ego-related addictions that is very common. To place oneself in the position of the judge means that the judge can have an opinion about everyone else but does not get judged themselves. Once again, it is an issue of power over others that can be used to feed the ego of the judge. There is also an inherent fear of losing the power over others when a judge consistently takes the position of being critical of everything around themselves. This could again be an overcompensation for experiencing a lack of power at some point in their personal history.

For addictions of intelligence, we often see a gravitation to anything that stimulates the intellectual mind. The greater the complexity of the explanations and concepts, the more one's self worth is fed. The ability to understand and implement complicated tasks that require intellect becomes the baseline for any solution. One example is the common perception that German automobiles are highly engineered, and thus of greater value. The flip side is that greater complexity of machines usually leads to greater chances of breakdown. Despite this higher likelihood of unreliability, the German automobile identity still tends toward a more highly engineered and complex solution being better.

Conversely, one can also be addicted to being weak and powerless, especially when doing so brings us something else that we need—usually attention, sympathy, or help of some other type. Once again, this is a situation where the root cause is not addressed, and the idea of inhabiting the weakness and powerlessness becomes a fabric of their container.

In other cases, our addictions may address the issue of overcompensation for one or more pivotal learning experiences in our lives. I recall a personal friend who was addicted to separation; in other words, the opposite of contact and connection. He would drift off in the middle of a conversation into an alternate world where he was in his element and fully in control. This inherently made it difficult to communicate as the idea of contact was untenable. After much deep discussion, I soon realized that he had verbally abusive parents who argued often and minimized his importance. Their arguments distressed him greatly as a child, and he developed an ability to "tune out" the discord and go to a safe place within his imagination at will. He was so good at moving back and forth between his physical state and imaginary world that you could barely sense a shift of attention in the middle of conversations. This affected him deeply as he was never truly deep in any conversation, and many of his relationships remained superficial.

Science in general is drawn to the idea of the "clean" study where the variable of interest is well isolated and confounding factors are easily controlled. This is inherently difficult when dealing with the multiple overlapping reasons for addiction. When we look at the current information available, the complexity of addiction becomes apparent as it is a multi-layered malfunction of normal neural systems. In essence, the normal mechanisms and machinery by which we learn, remember, emote, feel pleasure, and motivate ourselves is rewired for the purpose of attaining a high. It hijacks the survival mechanism of salience to place the addiction at the head of the priority list and conditions us to crave it with increasing intensity.

Addictions begin with the rewards centers being stimulated outside its normal environmental circumstances. It then changes the very basis of our genetic structure (epigenetic changes), inducing increased methylation of the DNA, a method by which a methyl group ($-CH_3$) is added to the DNA molecule. This process represses the activation of certain genes, effectively turning them off. In doing so, the normal controls to the expression of specific genes are disrupted. The extent of disruption is not entirely known, as gene expression changes can be very subtle. Some of these changes are thought to contribute to age-related pathologies, such as cancer, osteoarthritis, and neurodegeneration.[81] Clearly, these impairments co-opt normal regulatory functions, and disrupts them to create as yet unknown con-sequences. It is, however, known that these epigenetic changes can be passed down into offspring.[82] If we add the social-psychological dynamics of guilt and shame into this equation, the situation quickly snowballs into a quite complex dysfunction.

These are some of the instances where recognizing the pattern of behavior will allow you to alter patient behavior away from damaging and deleterious habits. If an instance of arrested development impedes progress in a health goal, we will need to probe to see if a patient is open to both bringing awareness to the root cause and addressing the ensuing damage.

For all manner of people suffering from addictions, Barbara O'Dair[83] in a Time Magazine Special Edition stated the dilemma of addiction succinctly: "whatever their compulsion is, it long ago stopped being fun." Whether it be a buzz or the relaxing effect of a drug or a drink, it is usually the feeling of the first hit that sends a person into a euphoric high. However, upon repeated use, the body begins to adapt and builds up tolerance to the drug, chemical, or behavior. Increasingly greater amounts are then needed to replicate the feeling of that first experience. At some point, the feeling of well-being and happiness of the first time diminishes and slowly begins to be replaced by the craving and desperation to return to the high. The process of going from the first euphoric experience to the distress of seeking more and more drugs evokes the accelerated transition of a young and inexperienced teenager to that of an old curmudgeon. Many have noted the accumulated effects of addiction leading to premature aging. The experience of addiction likens a microcosm of major life transition. It is no surprise that the native tribes of the Amazonian rain forest refer to their sacred and highly addictive medicinal ayahuasca as the "vine of the little death." It is highly likely that the indigenous Amazonian tribes knew quite a bit more about addiction than they have been given credit.

Along my journeys, it was not uncommon to run across Westerners who sought healing from shamans in the jungles of South America after being prescribed anti-psychotic and sedative medications by their medical doctors. What was apparent to me was that many were scarred from their experiences and were left with such a monumental feeling of distrust and anger that complicated their initial illnesses.

The idea of balance appeared to be a mirage that seemed simple enough yet was always tantalizingly out of reach. Yet in their eyes, I saw a glimmer of hope in the idea that balancing their internal emotional needs along with the elimination of the medications that dulled their senses was beginning the heavy work of rearranging the internals of their psyche.

The treatment of addiction has confounded modern medicine in many ways. Traditional medicine has fared marginally better. However, it is one area where modern medicine has adapted traditional techniques extensively, as seen in drug rehabilitation retreats. When examining the programs available at these facilities, a grab-bag of traditional methods like yoga, meditation, acupuncture, and intensive counseling therapy are commonplace. Yet one of the main treatments for opioid addiction (e.g. heroin, oxycodone, hydroxycodone) remains the replacement of the opioid with a slightly less addictive methadone.

When looking at the traditional healing of the ayahuasca shamans, we must give significant credit to the extensive amount of time spent prior to the ayahuasca ceremony. While there are variations in the preparation methods between shamans, this period can last for months. It begins with a prescribed cleansing that can include regular medicinal washings, a severely restricted diet, meditation, self-reflection, and counseling-like discussions. These are considered preparations under the guidance of the ayahuasca spirit. The therapy sessions trace the entire course of the patient's addiction, all the way back to the specific psychological needs that were seemingly filled by their object of addiction. It concentrates on the broken relationships that the addiction causes, and the subsequent pain that it inflicts. In magnifying the suffering of their personal relationships and acknowledging the impending diminishing high sensations experienced by the patient, the shaman lays out the framework of their projected downfall. The patient is given a choice to reach out for the help of the ayahuasca spirit, or to continue down the road of addiction. To my eyes, this entire preparation period infuses the patient with awareness of their own essential needs and belief in the powers of the medicine. The time spent on preparation allowed the patient to settle into a new routine, and deeply implant the idea of healing into their subconscious minds through the long-term memory.

This period of preparation has been mostly bypassed in modern medicine. Although it is somewhat mirrored in the emphasis on the first 90 days of treatment in twelve-step recovery programs, they spend significantly less time in preparation, and usually attempt to complete the in-house treatment phase within 30 days. While one month seems like a long time to busy people, it is barely adequate to establish a new routine into the long-term memory. The U.S. military branches have long used between 10-13 weeks for basic training (boot camp) partly for this reason. Admirably, current addiction treatment centers emphasize balance, yet the initial indoctrination is curtailed possibly due to financial constraints. Unfortunately, modern medicine is still lacking in the awareness and belief criteria.

CHAPTER 18

Constructive Envisioning *and* Fantasy

I n the course of dealing with patients as well as in daily social interactions, one of the common problems we face involves illusions created by people. At its inception, a simple "flight of fancy" is so named due to the leap of faith necessary in suspending the need to be grounded in reality. We have all at some point entertained ideas that appealed to us and placed ourselves into hypothetical situations. The presence of active fantasies in psyches are within variations of normal. Indeed, some temporary illusions are part of the process of envisioning a future that is desired, accounting for much of the creativity and technological advances in our modern world. It is even quite common for these illusions to set the stage for medical treatments.

Several years ago, Ben, an elderly male patient, insisted on recreating his smile from his teenage years. Never mind that he was in his early seventies with a history of gum recession and heavy dental wear due to work stress and multiple divorces. He had grown a long mustache and beard over the years in order to cover up his degrading teeth and gums. Upon his expression of general melancholy, I scrutinized his word choice to find that the early death of several of his closest friends triggered in him a period of deep self-reflection. In his newfound mindset, his teeth were the most visible part of him that required a reset and renewal. As his smile became unrecognizable in the mirror, he finally reached out to his general dentist to consider a dental reconstruction. Ben had been referred to me for gum grafting procedures to fill the dark spaces between his teeth. At the time, I remember being quite amused by his insistence on using his high school graduation photo as his envisioned outcome. I openly wondered about what he was truly seeking by presenting such an obviously dated photograph of himself. This led to my line of questioning that invoked a quiet contemplation in Ben.

However, his seriousness convinced me that we needed to discuss the limitations of gum grafting for certain types of gum recession. Over time, he became aware of what was physically possible as well as what was impossible with current technology. Through multiple appointments over two years, his general dentist and I coordinated our treatments to deliver a reconstruction of both his gums and teeth. In this case, we had to moderate and rebalance Ben's vision to what was physically possible.

In other cases, there is a point at which illusions cross the threshold of "normal." While some illusions are considered harmless machinations of a creative mind, others become intertwined with negative projections on the people around them. In short, illusions that are out of balance bypass the realm of reason into delusions.

When faced with a physical reality that does not match with their ideas of themselves and ego, minds can become disillusioned. In some instances, it can create an alternate perspective that allows them to keep feeding the perceived needs. In the event of disillusionment, we find the same classic stages involved in grief and loss: denial, anger, bargaining, depression, and eventually acceptance. The quicker these stages are cycled through, the more rapid the adaptation to the new situation becomes. When dealing with those who never reach acceptance, a created fantasy allows the person to maintain their course despite all physical signs pointing away from their delusion.

Many of the delusions in health deal with a refusal to accept the medical recommendations regardless of the scientific evidence upon which it was based. While "reality" may differ slightly based on the perspective of the viewer, it is not unusual to see elements of reality mixed into entire worlds of fantasy. In essence, the illusion that is created may be a skewed perception of something that is peppered with occasional facts. It is not uncommon for patients to fight recommendations to stop smoking or to eat more vegetables and fewer cookies. The eternal hope is that these patients will eventually come around. Yet until they do, it may be easier to avoid doctor visits than to be faced with the popping of their delusional bubble.

In a wider sense, the extent that social media companies have reached into reporting false news has set the stage for a version of mass delusion. It has never been easier to find some source, credible or not, that supports a patient's existing opinion and allows the continuation of the fantasy. As such, verification of any opinion can be found by way of Internet search engine.

Unfortunately, the advertisement of particular medications has become such a problem in modern medicine. Across the Internet, television, and radio, we often see and hear various medications advertised, to be followed by a long list of side effects in small print. Invariably, these commercials end with the phrase, "Ask your doctor about [insert brand name of drug]." Patients then proceed to look up information from the Internet that supports their hope that the drug can cure their affliction. The allure of the magical pill that fixes all their problems is as enduring as the snake oil of old. If they ever make it into a doctor's office, much of an appointment is spent sorting through all the misinformation found by the patient during their research. Much of this is the patient hearing what they want to hear without any fact checking.

As a background to this problem, we can trace this to the formative years of the Internet when various laws were passed in the United States,

Europe, and Australia that protected Internet companies from being sued for nonfactual material that was posted on their forums. In the United States, the Communications Decency Act was passed in 1996. A key portion of this law, Section 230, deemed that "interactive computer services" cannot be held as the publisher or speaker of third-party content.[84] While Section 230 is considered vital for preserving online free speech, it has also sheltered social media companies from lawsuits for slander, libel, and any false content masquerading as factual news. Pseudonyms and fabricated online identities also made it more difficult to identify the third-party source of the misinformation materials. As an increasing number of people look online for their information and news, their sense of normal can be easily manipulated based on control of the content. The resulting illusion bypasses the need for physical proof and becomes more reliant on the created fantasy. The normal feedback mechanism is checked by the need for verifiable physical proof.

Given proper verification, the illusion never gets past being a passing flight of fancy. Credible news agencies record their sources and devote resources to vetting them. Companies that serve as news aggregates, often lump the reputable news agencies directly beside the uncredited and anonymous sources. Despite collecting and peddling unvetted "news" reports, these companies are legally shielded by Section 230. Left to their own devices, this continues to feed unhealthy delusions. Unfortunately, the polarization will continue on its current course as long as what purports to be "news" is not held to a factual journalistic standard.

When examining the psychology that supports the creation of fantasies, a backstop of verifiable facts must be established. Upon departure from this model of verifiable proof, the left brain is removed from the equation. In its absence, the right brain creates a new reality to compensate for the loss of the left brain. The imagination takes on the central role in creating a fantasy to fit the model that no longer is attached to reality. In colloquial speech, the tail wags the dog.

One other critical step in reconnecting with people who carry delusions is the identification of their currency. What carries the highest priority and value in their fantasy? In Ben, it was the feeling of being young and attractive again. That was the root of the issue, rather than the expense of reconstructive dental procedures. His general dentist and I were able to reach him by empowering his reasonable illusions and providing him concrete short-term to long-term goals.

Recognize that the greater the rejection of proof, the further the imagination has to fill the void. The moment that the left brain is subdued, we see the right brain compensate. At the moment, we do not have a standardized evaluation of where the threshold stands between a simple flight of fancy (as we all have experienced in our childhood and adolescent development) and the beginning of mental disease. With multiple separate worlds of fantasy, we will start to see the chronic breakdown of the logical left brain. If one is unable to recover, we begin to see symptoms of multiple personalities and schizophrenia.

As healthcare guides to our patients, it is left to us to identify whether an initial illusion brought in by a patient has enough merit for us to empower it into a guiding vision. If indeed reality fails to support the illusion, we must dispel it such that it cannot grow into an out-of-control fantasy.

CHAPTER 19

Dealing *with* Phobias

In dentistry, we witness phobias on a widespread level much more than the general public. Webster's Dictionary describes a phobia as "an exaggerated, usually inexplicable, and illogical fear of a particular object, class of objects, or situation." In our terms, it takes the effect of a lesson learned so well that it makes its way into our subconscious mind. It is an experience which so overwhelmed the person that the object of phobia jumped the line into first priority whenever it is encountered.

As mentioned before, a sensitive-type person will be more likely to reach sensory overload at which point a phobia will be ingrained directly into the subconscious mind. It has been demonstrated that phobias can also stem from a non-experiential standpoint, meaning that it can be learned as well. In both cases, the fear mechanism in phobias are developed once the coping mechanisms are exhausted, and simple physical avoidance is not possible.[85] Due to the extreme fear involved in phobias, the amygdala, seat of the fight-or-flight response and primitive part of the brain, is strongly suspected of orchestrating the response.[86] As one of the most evolutionarily primitive parts of the brain, any phobia trigger leads to the immediate prioritization through the salience mechanism. Of course, time and regular replay of the trauma help magnify and ingrain the need to avoid a similar circumstance.

One obvious example (for me) would be a dental phobia. At some point, there was an initial exposure to a dentist that so overwhelmed the patient that a severe complex of avoidance was established in the subconscious mind. It is also possible that this fear can be established from hearing multiple horror stories of dental experiences. While phobias can develop at any point in a person's lifetime, those that occur in childhood seem to have a more profound effect even decades later. Typically, childhood experiences are exacerbated by the relative powerlessness of the child compared with the authoritative adult. The saying "once stung, twice shy" applies to this situation perfectly. When replayed over and over again, it is indeed a lesson deeply learned through repetition.

Whether the phobia stemmed from a personal experience or was a learned response, we can begin to unravel the trained reaction by offering an alternate possibility that does not include the feared trauma. The goal is for the patient to relearn a response that follows a different script than that of the phobia. Here is where our understanding of memory can assist in deemphasizing the fear and strengthening the memory of the positive aspects. We are essentially working to rewire the association of the activity with the fear, thus removing the response of fight-or-flight from the primitive portion of the brain. The repetition of a new script (a positive outcome, instead of the feared one) will over time replace parts of the phobia within the fabric of the container. For example, a common fear of needles is well embedded for many patients. As many healthcare practitioners are aware, most of the pain is not from the needle prick, but rather from the push of the plunger when the fluid displaces volume under the skin. In this case, constant contact and reassurance combined with slowing down the injection usually dramatically improves the experience.

In adding positive data points for the patient's recall of a past trauma, we are helping them remember the situation differently. We may never decouple the conditioning of aversion to pain, but if we can reassociate the experience with the benefits and disempower the irrational fear, we will have done the patient a great service. While the phobic patient may never completely unlearn the traumatic scenario, we can hope to establish a situation where the power of the phobia is reduced to a manageable level. This has been noted as one of the more common reasons given for appointment cancellations and no shows in dental offices. If the patient is able to complete a necessary dental procedure without losing sleep the night before and experiencing a dread of the appointment weeks ahead, then we have at least been able to minimize the negative outcome.

Much like cases of drug addiction, phobias demonstrate signs of dysfunction in the excessive stimulation of what otherwise are basic necessary pathways. It appears that each subsequent exposure of a phobia triggers an upregulation of the entire pathway to the amygdala. Similarly, each time an addictive drug is used, the reward pathways actually increase in strength due to an increase in dopamine receptors. The repetition of both these pathways leads to an increasingly severe fear in phobias and increasing high in drugs. In the case of phobias, D-cycloserine, a "sedative" for the amygdala, has shown some promise in decreasing the severity of phobias in children.[87]

At this juncture, the question arises of how much of the emotional side of healing is actually just forgetting the pain of the trauma? Herein lies one of the most commonly experienced yet least often discussed aspects of healing. The fading negative memory of the trauma needs to be balanced with something positive on the side of the particular activity involved or the healing itself. In other words, a lingering trauma inadvertently becomes a part of the container of the person, and there is an inherent replacement of something that used to be positive (the joys of whichever activity the person was engaged in at the time of the trauma) with the pain of the trauma. When this trauma becomes part of the container, a conscious decision on the part of the wounded person to remove it from the inside of container will be necessary in order to recover fully. The medical professional will be in a unique position to offer this awareness to the patient and can certainly assist in beginning the process of replacing the trauma with something positive and fulfilling. Over time, the complete replacement of the aforementioned trauma with the joy or love of the activity prior to the accident will constitute full emotional healing.

CHAPTER 20

Ego-Related Imbalances

While there are an infinite number of issues that can be rebalanced, there are a number of instances that are more common than others. When we deal with the motivations that lead us to make certain decisions, our idea of self often determines our choices. Why does someone make a choice that we may not? It entirely depends on their perspective and what priorities they have at the specific moment. As previously stated, our idea of self has been described as a container. Essentially, we are the container itself. We can decide what to place inside of the container, and what remains on the outside. We can also decide to remove something from the inside and replace it with something else. The choice of what to include and exclude is ours to make, and the idea of self will change as we learn both about the external world around us as well as the internal aspect within us. We are composed of all the programs and learned lessons and ideas of morality. The stronger our ego, the stronger the walls that separate the internal from the external aspects of the container.

There are instances when we value that which is inside our container much more than all the things and ideas that we chose to keep outside. This all-or-nothing approach feeds into the ego imbalances that can become a problem. In asserting the primacy of the things that we hold within our container, we in turn devalue everything that we excluded.

While this view is not always absolute, it becomes quite apparent to others when the ego is out of balance. When we assume that something has no value because it did not work for us, it undervalues all the possibilities that we have not yet considered. There is a natural judgment involved in determining what we choose for ourselves and its suitability for our own situation. However, when we extend that judgment beyond our own sphere of influence (basically anything that we can hope to affect an immediate change), there is an extension of perceived control assumed over someone else. In most societies, we describe this extension of control over others as *power*.

Recognize that power can be given by those who allow control over their own decisions or taken by those that make decisions for others. This has been a constant throughout recorded human existence and will likely remain so for the foreseeable future. The idea of power and where we stand in relation to it has been and is a struggle for many. Those who normally feel powerless may revel in the elevation of choice. Likewise those who are used to being in charge will expect to always be able to make their own choices. Conflicts in power begin when one individual or group regularly assumes the position for making the decisions for those who have not willingly given them that power. Those in power often easily forget that upon assuming their power, they can also be depriving others of their own personal choices.

There is another important aspect of our learning experience that must be addressed: the push-pull motivation dichotomy, otherwise known as the carrot versus the stick. Lindsey Agness, in her book *Change Your Life with NLP: The Powerful Way to Make Your Whole Life Better with Neuro-Linguistic Programming*,[88] discussed some of the factors in motivations seen in people. She describes "push motivation" as the impetus for change that "gets the ball rolling," is shorter acting, more reactive and emotionally based. In many cases, the push often centers on avoidance of perceived pain. Based on our model of mental structure, the push is emanating from the subconscious mind, and is carried through into the conscious. You may think of this as a fear-based motivator. As my graduate residency instructors used to opine, there are few motivators more compelling than fear. Considering the concept of fear triggering the fight-or-flight response, it serves to activate the amygdala, an evolutionarily ancient part of the brain. Conversely, "pull motivation" is based on being drawn to a concept or envisioned outcome. The pull exhibits a more sustained motivation, and is generally based on a positive, self-affirming feeling. In our model, the pull begins from the conscious mind, and then delves into the subconscious. Healer Karl Direske, who has been teaching this concept for well over a decade, describes this dichotomy as "pressure and tension." These are the fundamental impetuses that are both useful for affecting change within our lives.

There is indeed a preference in how different children accept information while the free will is not yet fully developed. As a matter of observation, this push-pull idea extends well into adulthood, and may be seen in different degrees throughout the lifetime. Some children seem to accept information being taught to them better if they are drawn to learn it by an incentive, whereas others will respond in a similar fashion if pressured by a negative stimulus.

For example, my son is most efficiently motivated when there is a positive incentive and an explicit perceived benefit to himself. He has always responded best to this manner of encouragement even in his infancy. There is an inherent wish to be inspired by something or someone great and wonderful to his young mind. Searching for the knowledge of what may be sufficient stimulus to draw him to action is a basic need for him and others like him.

On the other hand, my daughter thrives under the push or pressure. I may give her a nudge to do a project with the implication of someone else beating her to the finish, and her motivation is direct and concentrated. She has a natural fear of my disapproval, much like many daughters, even if I do not outwardly show disappointment in her choices. If there is a deadline, she will increase her speed and productivity in whatever task to rise to the occasion. The fear of failure and loss of something dear to her sends her into a work ethic that shames even most adults.

There is something intensely personal about these different approaches that centers on how people see themselves and the development of their egos. The fundamental difference is quite dramatic, and we can observe this dichotomy clearly in both the general public as well as patients that arrive in need of our expertise and care. It is important to accept that both these processes individually and in combination will allow a person to affect a change in their lives. Neither is inherently superior or inferior to the other, although reflectively, the pull seems to have greater longevity when effecting long term goals.

Most accomplished professionals will likely have extensive training in development of their egos, as they have been through the rigors of setting and achieving multiple goals, which naturally builds confidence. As such, our society favorably selects those who are strong in ego. In fact, it is quite necessary to achieve success in life. This in turn also may influence the population that tends to seek regular healthcare. A well-developed ego may be one of the strongest assets to many of our patients. In addressing this type of imbalance, we need only to increase awareness of the downstream effects of decisions made and their unintended consequences. Taking care to frame the presented options in a way that preserves some choice for them will be key.

In situations of the under-developed ego, we will witness much self-doubt, difficulty in making decisions, and regular ceding of power to others. These are circumstances in which the walls of the container are barely existing, and what goes in and what stays out can be easily manipulated. More time will be necessary in dealing with these situations as there is much difficulty is building upon previous decisions. In fact, the decision tree may be undermined at every branch. When encountering these cases, we can gain ground by emphasizing the communication from the subconscious mind. The subconscious mind has already sorted through the multitude of sensory and intellectual inputs and has given the overall assessment in the gut feeling. Make extensive note of the feelings of a person who is experiencing an ego deficit. You may need to replay these communications back to the patient and reinforce what their subconscious is already telling them.

For the purposes of bedside manner and healing, we want to minimize use of this influence over a patient's choice, unless they specifically request our personal opinion. Some will feel empowered by being given a choice, while others will feel burdened. When we take that step to influence the decisions of others, we may inadvertently assume responsibility for that decision in the mind of the patient. Whether the patient sees this as a benefit or liability will depend on the patient and their view of success. If we are able to frame the options and fully inform our patient of the benefits and disadvantages (as ethically required in informed consent), we can ensure the patient's participation in responsibility for themselves.

We will naturally have an assessment and judgment of any situation or treatment course. Our judgment must be tempered with the thought that the variables of our individual circumstances are so vast that differences in method, path, and goals between ourselves and our patients are inevitable. We can still value what has worked well for us yet retain other options for future consideration. Herein lies the critical nature of being in balance in our own lives.

There appears to be a natural blind spot in our awareness that includes most of our own deficiencies. This is likely for self-preservation purposes as our ego may not survive if we delved into all our faults and imbalances simultaneously. This blind spot results from the fine line between constructive criticism, which is meant as feedback and a pathway for improvement, as opposed to an attack, meant to break down and diminish. The main difference between the constructive criticism and an attack is the contact created when you establish the ability to relate to the other person involved. It is important to leave our judgments at the door for both our patients as well as ourselves in these assessments. As difficult as it may be, we also must be completely truthful to ourselves when becoming aware of our own biases. Whereas it is preferable to address and improve in areas where we are deficient, it may not be expedient or even possible on the short term. Acknowledging these individual idiosyncrasies will allow us to work around them and still maintain functionality. A neutral frame of mind is essential to gain this awareness.

It is very helpful to have others around us who are also going through the process of neutralizing our own deficiencies. This brings up the idea of increasing the training circle to those working with us (assistants, technicians, nurses, and other hands-on medical professionals) in these concepts so that we can have a check and balance on our assessments. When seen through the lens of someone else we trust, we are also more likely to listen and hear something that may otherwise be very difficult to accept.

There is an enormously powerful connection formed when we witness another person dealing with an issue with which we have personal experience. We may have a uniquely visceral memory of how we dealt with our situation—whether successfully or unsuccessfully. However, we must realize that each case is unique and may have a different dynamic which may require a different solution. What worked for us personally may not work for others. For example, if we see a person suffering from cancer, we may draw from our own experience with other cancer patients or possibly even our own personal experience with the disease. The manner in which we acquired the disease (e.g. environmental exposure vs. genetic predisposition) may be completely different and thus will require their own unique treatment path. The fact that our destination may be similar does not mean that we could not have taken different paths to get there.

The patient's experience resonates with that of our own within the walls of our container.

The better we know ourselves, the more likely we will be able to see our own strengths and deficiencies. Are our own egos in check, or do they actually work against us? Are we treating strictly the concerns of the patient, or are we somewhat addressing our own needs in the process? There are many instances where I have realized that my suggested treatment for a patient also will apply to something within my own personal life. It is the reason and the connection that allowed me to relate to the specific patient and their problem. In a sense, it is a problem that we both share, thus making the solution a joint success. In these instances, should we insist on a particular course of treatment for a patient, we must be mindful of whether we are treating our own concerns or strictly those of our patient.

If we lack in our personal balance, our awareness is hampered, and we may not recognize that when we deprive our patients of choice, we deprive them of their sense of self. This is contrary to our idea of healing and "restoring the whole" and must be avoided at all costs.

CHAPTER 21

Putting It All Together

Throughout our discourse, we have visited several healing traditions that highlighted our key commonalities. However, there are many more throughout the world that are no less compelling and fascinating. Ayurvedic medicine, rooted in India from the Bronze Age, and then codified from the fourth to sixth centuries CE, is another traditional healing method that exemplifies our crucial elements. To the Maori people of New Zealand and Oceania, we once again see the same elements to their traditional ideas of health. In fact, nearly every culture that has a healing role for shaman has exhibited these qualities.

In his instant classic, simply titled *Shamanism*, Michael Winkelman linked together the criteria shared among shamanic groups worldwide, to shed light on the use of various states of altered consciousness to create the awareness necessary for both hindsight and foresight.[89] He weaves a web that stretches between the historical origins of shamanism to the current understanding of how the phenomenon is necessary to feed the biological, psychological, and sociological needs of human societies. Among his arguments is the role of the shaman as healer.

From personal observations, I find that my criteria for healing runs remarkably consistent when viewed in the same light as they are based on the similarities in the basic biology and consciousness of all humanity. Beyond the confines of "noble savages" on one end, and "underdeveloped children" on the other, indigenous peoples have the same complexity and depth of character that all humans have as we struggle with life and its meaning. Time and again, the same principles and themes reach out to us across the ages. It seems as if these traditions from all around the world speak to us, breaching the veils of time, space, and centuries of wounding to embrace our common humanity.

In identifying the three elements of awareness, belief, and balance in the context of healing, we begin to realize that they exist prominently in every healing modality the world over, with the notable exception of Western medicine. There is a synergistic effect when these three criteria are brought together. Awareness by itself is purely information, passive in its nature, and incapable of affecting change. Belief on its own can easily be a fantasy. Awareness and belief together (without balance) could be a subtext to a horror movie. Balance alone is seen as both submissive and resigned and has been pushed aside in the name of progress for much of modern times. In the popular consciousness, it was not until George Lucas brought back the idea of balance (in the Force) in his fictional Star Wars saga that the general public was reintroduced to this concept.

When we align awareness, belief, and balance in sequence together, we arrive at a formula that speaks to us through the fabric of our fundamental building blocks. While modern medicine may inadvertently dabble in some aspects of our three elements, we have not expressly stated these criteria as our goals. So often do we assume that science automatically elicits belief in our patients. Has our scientific and technological emphasis led us to stray from one of the basic sets of requirements for complete healing of the mind, body, and spirit? More importantly, can we reintegrate something so fundamental back into our medical systems?

When we look at the depressed, downtrodden, and nonresponsive outliers to our modern treatments, should we consider that there is something missing in our current model of health? According to the research of

Tommy Begay, cultural psychologist at the University of Arizona College of Medicine, reintroducing elements of Navajo culture back into health services in Navajo Nation has a significant positive effect on sleep-related cardiovascular and metabolic disease.[90] He noted the established link between poor sleep and apnea with heart conditions and poor diabetes control. The reintroduction of "belief" back into the public health equation appeared to support improvements in sleep especially where other treatments were not effective.

A number of years ago, the late comparative mythologist Joseph Campbell studied a vast breadth of world mythologies and literature to isolate the universal need for certain elements in our heroes. Here we are asking a similar question, but in a slightly different vein. What does the need for these three elements—expanding awareness, cultivating belief, and establishing and maintaining balance—say about us as a species? Are we somehow looking at a time-tested method to reestablish the peace, love, joy, and purpose that we so desperately seek? Can we restore a missing ingredient to return the soul to modern medicine? These are anything but rhetorical questions to be tended to at our convenience.

The application of awareness and belief allow us as healers to access our patients and perform our treatments. This gets us in the door, so to speak. However, it is the balance portion that guides our treatment and sets the stage for long term sustainability and health. We are balancing ideas, lifestyles, and perceptions. Typically, we can see the big picture view of patients' health in a way they cannot. They may not necessarily like the rebalancing especially if they are accustomed to the imbalance. Some resistance is expected, yet when the long-term rebalancing bears fruit, our patients will feel the improvement.

Our patients and people we interact with during daily activities will exhibit all the elements of mental development that we have covered over the course of this book—a final review of core lessons to keep in mind might be helpful.

Should we recognize a pattern in a patient, sometimes the urge to divulge our observations comes to the forefront. It is important to give people the freedom and opportunity to work out their own issues. Unsolicited advice is typically unwelcome.

While it may not necessarily change treatment recommendations drastically, we will need to account for patient threshold. This threshold will apply to sensitivity, coping ability, and capacity to directly address the root issues. What is the difference between two individuals who are subjected to similar stresses, but one suffers from PTSD and the other remains resilient? Spotting the patients who are coping well with challenges versus those that are beyond their threshold and overwhelmed will be a critical factor in connecting and communicating effectively. Sometimes, an individual will already be at the limit of their threshold upon initial presentation. This may be one of the main criteria on determining the appropriate time to refer a patient for mental health treatment. Along these lines, recognize that the ability to cope changes over a lifetime. Even in normal development, a person will cope with some difficulties, and be wounded by others. The mental and physical scars that we bear ultimately play a large role in developing our individual personalities. Without these considerations, we will only be treating the disease but neglecting the patient as a whole.

Cognitive reframing can be used in a variety of situations from simply suggesting a different perspective and resetting the goalposts to intensively deprogramming the dysfunctional circuits reinforced through chemical or behavioral addiction. It can also be used to replace destructive habits with healthy ones.

As in most of our lives, the daily fatigue, responsibilities, and the progress on our mental checklists will play a role in our awareness as well as that of our patients. Our daily burdens contribute to the baseline of stress that can alter the sensitivity and coping threshold significantly throughout the day. There are moments when patients are both awake and cognitively processing at a peak and will be most receptive to complex treatment plans and other intellectual discourse. In the remainder of the situations, fatigue and stress may blunt their capacity for eloquent verbal communication. These are the situations when reading body language and altering your approach to ease the strain on your patients will be greatly appreciated.

Coming back to our recurring practical example, we find that Ella has completed dental treatment successfully. Her self-esteem is much improved, particularly due to her efforts in reducing weight and controlling diabetes. Her internist had been working with her to relearn the basics of practical nutrition and exercise. She has learned how to choose her foods considering the glycemic index (blood glucose levels), balance the healthy foods with occasional snacks, and has begun exercising on a regular basis. She has gained positive new relationships through a hiking club and ceased smoking as her overall stress has improved. She clearly has incorporated the new information and structure into her daily routine, thus bringing overall balance back into her life. It was her choice to embark on a new healthier path. Our teamwork along with all her other health advisors were able to equip her with the necessary guidance to achieve her goals. Continued support will be critical for long-term success as she is susceptible to relapse in smoking and depression if she hits a rough patch. Of course, Ella is but one type of patient and represents one of the more satisfying instances. Often, our successes are not so spectacular and complete, and we may need to repeat certain lessons and treatments. We may be dealing with multitudes of partial successes and failures. It is these fragmentary wins and losses that form the lens through which we view our professions and our lives.

Throughout training and in private practice, there is a rough structure to the interactions that make up an appointment with a healthcare practitioner. In many cases, this structure is an adequate means to render episodic treatment. Unfortunately, there are many instances in which it is not enough. Traditional medicine the world over has been used to great effect for many generations. In reexamining the traditional elements which are so central to a plethora of traditional medicinal practices, the three main categorical lessons of expanding awareness, cultivating belief, and establishing and maintaining balance arise. If we are able to embrace and integrate these lessons into our daily routines and utilize them as the foundation of the relationships with our patients, we may well be tapping into the very fabric of what it means to heal. It is my sincere belief that patient satisfaction will correspondingly increase.

CHAPTER 22

Future Directions

During the preparation of this manuscript, it has become all but impossible to neglect to the COVID-19 pandemic. It has altered our calculus on the balance between personal medicine and community medicine. The analysis of the performance of the medical systems in both China and Italy have accentuated the simultaneous need for both tracks.[91] The differences in approach between personal health and public health have never been more laid bare by the comparison between the two systems. The Italian system (remarkably similar to most western countries, including the United States) is based on quality personal care, while the Chinese medical system is skewed toward overall health for entire communities. More specific examples of quality personal care include expertise in complicated surgeries, transplants, sports medicine, and extensive life support, while public health deals with vaccinations, primary care, emergency room, pediatric, and preventive care.

While both medical systems were inundated with the sheer numbers of people needing care, the Italian system was especially compromised due to the prospective COVID-19 patients mixing with the non-infected patients while in the waiting rooms. As a result, healthcare workers and entire hospitals became vectors for the virus. In hindsight, segregating the COVID-19 patients from the rest of the hospital may have prevented some of the problems. Mirco Nacoti and his research group suggested reserving the hospital beds for the seriously ill, and establishing satellite clinics for testing and palliative care, along with access to telemedicine. The coronavirus has a unique characteristic of exploiting a weakness in community medicine (poor access to care, incomplete community-wide immunizations and vaccinations, providing essential healthcare services despite inability to pay). The differences in approach to health vary from location to location, but the systems with a majority component of socialized public health (South Korea, Vietnam, Taiwan, China, Australia, New Zealand, Iceland, Finland, Norway, Denmark, among others) seemed to have been better positioned to fight a disease like COVID-19. From cursory evaluations of healthcare systems worldwide, it is clear that we should not pit the private and community systems against each other but incorporate aspects of both.

Due to the specific need to protect healthcare workers, as well as isolation requirements for patients, the future for telemedicine has been all but assured. Despite my use of the initial failure of telemedicine as an example earlier in this book, I want to emphasize that in the Fremont case, the failure was not a technology failure but a human failure. Ultimately, it was the improper application of a public health tool on a very personal health problem. The goal of utilizing technology to enhance the patient experience is an admirable one based on the progression of science for the greater good. Like most tools, it is only as good as the person or group wielding the tool.

With that being said, the field of telemedicine has a great deal to gain from incorporation of the techniques described in this text. For obvious reasons, the use of telemedicine reduces the amount of information gathering that is accessible to the healthcare practitioner in the diagnosis phase. Connections are much more difficult to establish as well as to maintain through an audio-video feed. It can be similar to wearing blinders compared with the full range of tools available when in the physical presence of the patient. In addition, body language and physical cues cannot be expressed or read with the same level of connection. Fortunately, most patients already have this expectation when accessing telemedicine.

When we consider the challenges presented by the limitations on awareness, we must doubly make sure that our verbal communications are clear, concise, and without any confusion. Eye contact becomes especially important because you lose many of the body language cues over a video screen. Humor is still possible and would likely be as appreciated as in-person, considering the rationale for the use of telemedicine in that case (perhaps an isolation due to infection, or lack of another doctor in the physical area). The value of facial expressions is accentuated, while movements of the hands and legs will not be visible.

During the economic shutdowns in the United States, online clothing vendors noted a significant increase in the sale of upper body clothing, such as shirts, blouses, ties, and jackets, while the usually associated lower body accompaniment, i.e., pants, skirts, shoes, socks, sold in far fewer quantities. Trend watchers keenly noted that the lower body was not visible while on the camera for telecommuting or conference call type applications. If we consider the limited scope of the camera, we can appreciate that it unexpectedly emphasizes all the things that are visible. This is certainly the case for telemedicine, and the need for improvements in bedside manner will be magnified.

Yet telemedicine is but one new tool to help us achieve a healing-centered future. Estimates vary, but the increase in use of telemedicine is apparent during the COVID-19 pandemic. We need to do more than simply wield new tools—we need to take a step back and look at the entire toolbox with a new perspective. Enabling a shift in perspective is often the difference between viewing a treatment as a success or failure. A simple switch in viewpoint may be just the right medicine. In remembering the late Apple Computers cofounder Steve Jobs' commencement address to the graduating class of 2005 at Stanford University, I recall him speaking on the fear of death emanating from his cancer diagnosis. Spoken bluntly, "No one wants to die. Even people who want to go to heaven don't want to die to get there." We can all relate to the idea of loss in a premature death. At this point, the morbid perspective of losing everything in life dominates.

In processing the extent of medicine in curing his condition, he eventually took on a more philosophical approach. "Remembering that I'll be dead soon is the most important tool I've ever encountered to help me make the big choices in life. Because almost everything—all external expectations, all pride, all fear of embarrassment or failure—these things just fall away in the face of death, leaving only what is truly important. Remembering that you are going to die is the best way I know to avoid the trap of thinking you have something to lose. You are already naked. There is no reason not to follow your heart." As he began to embrace his inevitable death, this simple change in perspective allowed him to embrace living ever more fiercely.

This changing of perspectives is the shift we seek especially when dealing with unrealistic expectations. Managing a patient's expectation is best done prior to performing the treatment itself. If a patient is advised of reasonable expectations, the likelihood of it being perceived as "after the fact spin" decreases significantly. As such, the awareness and assessment of where you stand in the patient's eyes will give you a great deal of information with which to work. Being able to read where a person stands upon initial interaction with you will give you the necessary basic information to approach them in a friendly non-confrontational manner. In essence, it allows you to avoid any clash of personalities right off the bat. Personally, I have found it most beneficial to maintain a neutral stance and maintain that I am merely a guide for the patient in their journey to health. This removes the extreme feelings out of the credit and/or blame game. While there are absolute successes and morbidity rates, ultimately our ability to frame the treatment into a larger context will determine whether something is a done deal, or still a work in progress. For better or worse, this is one of the main reasons for satisfaction or dissatisfaction with a healthcare professional from the standpoint of a patient.

Let us emphasize the humanity in healthcare and raise the overall level of care by improving our communication and working on a very personal level in full support of our patient's best interest. Many of us have forgotten that which brings us together and the common thread that we all share. Recognizing that we are all "works in progress" allows the room for further communication. For those who are inclined, this deep integration of psychology into our everyday practice is the key to reaching the next level of premium healthcare. For those who merely wish to improve their business dealings, recognize that this same skill set is also the key to avoiding the unresolved disagreements that lead to lawsuits in our professions.

Recognize that this perspective allows us unparalleled clarity into the basis of communication. Every person possesses an inherent ability to determine whether an interaction is friendly or holds the threat of danger. In our approach, we can appeal to the positive aspects by making connections and affirming our commonalities, thus ensuring that we keep the interaction on the positive side. Conversely, miscommunications and detachment will send a threatening signal, to which most people will react with defensive behavior. This fight-or-flight response is quite conducive to overreaction and even violence. When we are able to control this initial approach to our daily interactions, we are actively appealing to the light side of everyone we encounter. These are skills that are central to the ability to hear and be heard clearly. In layman's terms, our topic may be casually described as bedside or chairside manner or ability to listen. However, as you have now become aware, it is not merely an intangible quality but instead a fully learnable and teachable subject and an essential soft skill for the current and next generations of healers.

Further development of this patient-centered approach to medicine is a critical next step in improving overall healthcare. Derived directly from careful analysis of the inner workings of our basic human psychology, it is this both novel and ancient approach that brings our attention back to the idea of personal medicine. As we are all patients at some point, we have a responsibility to push for the medical industry to address our particular needs. In the absence of this consumer pressure, the medical corporations will dictate to us what they think our needs should be. If you are a patient seeking a new healthcare practitioner, for example, testing the responsiveness of your prospective doctor as detailed in prior chapters may reveal how aware your doctor is to your needs. Elevating overall awareness to a major criterion in your search for the right doctor may be advisable. Indeed, every patient should have an expectation that their healthcare worker be familiar with these concepts. When the patient demands the change, a new standard will arise, benefiting the overall state of healthcare the world over.

From the lessons of the COVID-19 pandemic, it has become abundantly clear that we must make room for both personal and community-wide public health. Large institutions and hospitals will need to recognize and match the patient to their specific needs. When viewing the public as a patient, we must acknowledge the differences in "currency" among the many groups that make up our population. While science is one possible currency, faith, connection, personality, flexibility, and empathy can also be highly valued. The over-reliance on science as belief (and refusal to shift to another currency) can lead to a particularly strong emotional response from vast segments of society. In the tempest formed from the mainstream media demonizing differences in opinion, public health officials in the United States struggled mightily to communicate during the pandemic. The failure to engage the belief criterium was apparent. When our national divisions are placed into the context of the three key criteria for healing, the deficiencies are laid bare. The end result is and will always be fragmented compliance to medical advice.

In individual practices, the development of teams to directly amplify the incoming information will accelerate patient assessments. In other words, different people may individually pick up pieces of information that can then be assembled into a greater map of the patients internal and external concerns. The benefits of having a team approach are that you will likely be more receptive to the imbalance others see in you. You may separate the tasks between different individuals such that each person can look at a particular aspect with more sensitivity and greater degree of attention. For example, a person walking into an office may express particular feelings to a receptionist that they would never say to a doctor. The nurse may then take the vital signs and pick up further information about the patient's day and outlook on their illness. By the time a doctor or therapist comes into contact with the patient, there is already a basis of information with which to work. When working in groups, healthcare practitioners may be able to concentrate on particular areas of concern, and thus streamline the entire process of information gathering. This team approach will more effectively utilize the awareness of multiple persons who will have their own individual strengths and weaknesses. By collaborating in this manner, we can generate significantly greater data points to create the overall picture of health for any patient. A system of checks and balances can be established to maintain the point of fulcrum as an overall baseline. From the standpoint of a patient, this type of team gives the positive impression of a well-integrated orchestra working to its maximum potential in support of the ultimate goal of maximal health for the individual patient.

No matter the size of the hospital or practice, the importance of the initial assessment becomes even more pivotal to proper care. The same hospital that introduced the robot in Fremont has also been lauded for running an efficient two track system for dealing with previous influenza seasons. Public health and epidemiology are important for creation of appropriate policy for entire populations. Both personal and community-wide medicine serve a useful purpose within the framework of overall health in our country. We must press the issue in order to achieve a balance that best serves our most basic needs.

Training for bedside manner should be incorporated into all professional schools. Taking it another step further, selecting candidate students who are naturally predisposed to awareness would fundamentally move the needle towards greater patient responsiveness with all graduates. The capacity for empathy (based on Elaine Aron's assessment of sensitivity), emotional intelligence, and communicative development should be added as acceptance criteria. Only then will we ensure that all graduates have practical tools for success. The laser-focus necessary for academic success sometimes obscures the need for exceptional interactive skills. It is quite apparent that the criteria for a "good" doctor differs significantly between the patient versus that of the professor. Widening the scope of professional education to include training in soft skills will narrow this gap significantly.

Medicine should be the ultimate service industry as it is determined directly by our health needs. As the needs evolve, so should our medical system and approach. Let us reflect and refocus our efforts on personal medicine development. To this end, I only hope to have changed your perspective. When we look at the world of medicine with these new eyes, it may change nothing or it may change everything. What we do with that changed perspective will be the beginning of something new. Nothing less than our lives depend upon it.

BIBLIOGRAPHY

1   Bliss M. *William Osler: A Life in Medicine.* Oxford: Oxford University Press, 1999

2   Black Elk; Joseph Epes Brown. *The Sacred Pipe.* University of Oklahoma Press, 1953.

3   Low, Sam. *Hawaiki Rising: Hōkūleʻa, Nainoa Thompson, and the Hawaiian Renaissance.* Honolulu, University of Hawaiʻi Press, 2018 [2013]. 344 pp. ISBN 9780824877354

4   Sexton R, Stabbursvik EA. Healing in the Sámi North. *Cult Med Psychiatry.* 2010;34(4):571-589. doi:10.1007/s11013-010-9191-x

5   Lown B. *The Lost Art of Healing.* New York: Ballantine Books; 1996.

6   Epstein RM. Mindful practice. JAMA. 1999 Sep 1;282(9):833-9.

7   Luis Garcia-Ballester, Jon Arrizabalaga, Montserrat Cabré, Lluís Cifuentes. (2002) Galen and Galenism, Burlington: Ashgate-Variorum

8   Silverman BD. Physician behavior and bedside manners: the influence of William Osler and The Johns Hopkins School of Medicine. *Proc (Bayl Univ Med Cent).* 2012 Jan;25(1):58-61. doi: 10.1080/08998280.2012.11928784. PMID: 22275787; PMCID: PMC3246857.

9   Atkinson, R.C. and Shiffrin, R.M. (1968). 'Human memory: A Proposed System and its Control Processes'. In Spence, K.W. and Spence, J.T. *The psychology of learning and motivation,* (Volume 2). New York: Academic Press.

10 Tipper CM, Signorini G, Grafton ST. Body language in the brain: constructing meaning from expressive movement. *Front Hum Neurosci.* 2015;9:450. Doi:10.3389/fnhum.2015.00450

[11] Fodor, Jerry A. (1983). *Modularity of Mind: An Essay on Faculty Psychology.* Cambridge, Massachusetts: MIT Press. ISBN 0-262-56025-9

[12] Kenrick, D. T., & Griskevicius, V. (2013). *The rational animal: how evolution made us smarter than we think.* New York: Basic Books.

[13] Juliane Kaminski, Bridget M. Waller, Rui Diogo, Adam Hartstone-Rose, Anne M. Burrows. Evolution of facial muscle anatomy in dogs. *Proceedings of the National Academy of Sciences* Jul 2019, 116 (29) 14677-14681; DOI: 10.1073/pnas.1820653116

[14] Charlet A, Grinevich V. Oxytocin Mobilizes Midbrain Dopamine toward Sociality. *Neuron.* 2017 Jul 19;95(2):235-237. doi: 10.1016/j.neuron.2017.07.002.

[15] Gazzaniga MS. The split-brain: rooting consciousness in biology. *Proc Natl Acad Sci USA.* 2014;111(51):18093-4. doi: 10.1073/pnas.1417892111

[16] wildernessFusion Niasziih Healing School, www.wildernessfusion.com

[17] *Principles of Neural Science,* Fifth Editon. Eric R. Kandel, Editor, James H. Schwartz, Editor, Thomas M. Jessell, Editor, Steven A. Siegelbaum, Editor, A. J. Hudspeth, Editor, Sarah Mack, Art Editor

[18] Feld GB, Born J. Sculpting memory during sleep: concurrent consolidation and forgetting. *Curr Opin Neurobiol.* 2017 Jun;44:20-27. doi: 10.1016/j.conb.2017.02.012. Epub 2017 Mar 6.

[19] Wright, Robert. *The Moral Animal: Why we are the way we are: The New Science of Evolutionary Psychology.* 1st ed. New York, Pantheon, 1994

[20] Gladwell, Malcolm. *Outliers: The Story of Success.* 1st ed. New York: Little, Brown and Company, 2008.

[21] Nickerson, Raymond S. (June 1998), Confirmation bias: A ubiquitous phenomenon in many guises, *Review of General Psychology,* **2** (2): 175–220, doi:10.1037/1089-2680.2.2.175

22 Wang Y, McKee M, Torbica A, Stuckler D. Systematic Literature Review on the Spread of Health-related Misinformation on Social Media. *Soc Sci Med.* 2019 Sep 18;240:112552. doi: 10.1016/j. socscimed.2019.112552.

23 Brohan J, Goudra BG. The Role of GABA Receptor Agonists in Anesthesia and Sedation. *CNS Drugs.* 2017 Oct;31(10):845-856. doi: 10.1007/s40263-017-0463-7.

24 Liu M, Luo J. Relationship between peripheral blood dopamine level and internet addiction disorder in adolescents: a pilot study. *Int J Clin Exp Med.* 2015 Jun 15;8(6):9943-8. eCollection 2015.

25 Silk JS, Lee KH, Elliott RD, Hooley JM, Dahl RE, Barber A, Siegle GJ. 'Mom-I don't want to hear it': Brain response to maternal praise and criticism in adolescents with major depressive disorder. *Soc Cogn Affect Neurosci.* 2017 May 1;12(5):729-738. doi: 10.1093/scan/nsx014.

26 Gerhardt KJ, Abrams RM. Fetal exposures to sound and vibroacoustic stimulation. *J Perinatol.* 2000 Dec;20(8 Pt 2):S21-30.

27 Alberini CM, Travaglia A. Infantile Amnesia: A Critical Period of Learning to Learn and Remember. *J Neurosci.* 2017 Jun 14;37(24):5783-5795. doi: 10.1523/JNEUROSCI.0324-17.2017.

28 Bauer PJ, Larkina M. Childhood amnesia in the making: different distributions of autobiographical memories in children and adults. *J Exp Psychol Gen.* 2014 Apr;143(2):597-611. doi: 10.1037/a0033307. Epub 2013 Aug 12.

29 Bauer PJ. Constructing a past in infancy: a neuro-developmental account. *Trends Cogn Sci.* 2006 Apr;10(4):175-81. Epub 2006 Mar 14.

30 Teicher MH, Samson JA. Annual Research Review: Enduring neurobiological effects of childhood abuse and neglect. *J Child Psychol Psychiatry.* 2016 Mar;57(3):241-66. doi: 10.1111/jcpp.12507. Epub 2016 Feb 1. Review. PMID:26831814;

Bos KJ, Zeanah CH Jr, Smyke AT, Fox NA, Nelson CA 3rd. Stereotypies in children with a history of early institutional care. *Arch Pediatr Adolesc Med.* 2010 May;164(5):406-11. doi: 10.1001/archpediatrics.2010.47.

[31] Bauer PJ, Larkina M. The onset of childhood amnesia in childhood: a prospective investigation of the course and determinants of forgetting of early-life events. *Memory.* 2014;22(8):907-24. doi: 10.1080/09658211.2013.854806. Epub 2013 Nov 18.

[32] Rachel S. Herz. The Role of Odor-Evoked Memory in Psychological and Physiological Health. *Brain Sci.* 2016 Sep; 6(3): 22. Published online 2016 Jul 19. doi: 10.3390/brainsci6030022. PMCID: PMC5039451. PMID: 27447673

[33] Chris R. Brewin and Bernice Andrews. Creating Memories for False Autobiographical Events in Childhood: A Systematic Review. *Appl Cogn Psychol.* 2017 Jan-Feb; 31(1): 2–23. Published online 2016 Apr 8. doi: 10.1002/acp.3220. PMCID: PMC5248593. PMID: 28163368

[34] Mark L. Howe and Lauren M. Knott. The fallibility of memory in judicial processes: Lessons from the past and their modern consequences. *Memory.* 2015 Jul 4; 23(5): 633–656. Published online 2015 Feb 23. doi: 10.1080/09658211.2015.1010709. PMCID: PMC4409058. PMID: 25706242

[35] Hamer, Dean. *The God Gene: How Faith Is Hardwired Into Our Genes.* Anchor Books, 2005. ISBN 0-385-72031-9.

[36] D J McKenna, G H Towers, F Abbott. Monoamine oxidase inhibitors in South American hallucinogenic plants: tryptamine and beta-carboline constituents of ayahuasca. *J Ethnopharmacol.* 1984 Apr;10(2):195-223. doi: 10.1016/0378-8741(84)90003-5. PMID: 6587171. DOI: 10.1016/0378-8741(84)90003-5;
Savoldi R, Polari D, Pinheiro-da-Silva J, Silva PF, Lobao-Soares B, Yonamine M, Freire FAM, Luchiari AC. Behavioral Changes Over

Time Following Ayahuasca Exposure in Zebrafish. *Front Behav Neurosci.* 2017 Jul 28;11:139. doi: 10.3389/fnbeh.2017.00139. PMID: 28804451; PMCID: PMC5532431.

37 Strassman RJ, Qualls CR, Uhlenhuth EH, Kellner R. Dose-response study of N, N-dimethyltryptamine in humans: II. Subjective effects and preliminary results of a new rating scale. *Arch Gen Psychiatry.* 1994;51:98-108.

38 Riba J, Valle M, Urbano G, Yritia M, Morte A, Barbanoj MJ. Human pharmacology of ayahuasca: subjective and cardiovascular effects, monoamine metabolite excretion, and pharmacokinetics. *J Pharmacol Exp Ther.* 2003 Jul; 306(1):73-83.

39 Naranjo, Claudio (1974). *The Healing Journey.* Pantheon Books. pp. X. ISBN 9780394488264.

40 Riba J, Rodríguez-Fornells A, Urbano G, Morte A, Antonijoan R, Montero M, et al. Subjective effects and tolerability of the South American psychoactive beverage ayahuasca in healthy volunteers. Psychopharmacology (Berl). 2001;154:85-95; Martial C, Cassol H, Charland-Verville V, Pallavicini C, Sanz C, Zamberlan F, et al. Neurochemical models of near-death experiences: a large-scale study based on the semantic similarity of written reports. Conscious Cogn. 2019;69:52-69.

41 Hamill J, Hallak J, Dursun SM, Baker G. Ayahuasca: Psychological and Physiologic Effects, Pharmacology and Potential Uses in Addiction and Mental Illness. *Curr Neuropharmacol.* 2019;17(2):108-128. doi:10.2174/1570159X16666180125095902; Malcolm BJ, Lee KC. *Ayahuasca:* An ancient sacrament for treatment of contemporary psychiatric illness?. *Ment Health Clin.* 2018;7(1):39-45. Published 2018 Mar 23. doi: 10.9740/mhc.2017.01.039; Domínguez-Clavé E, Soler J, Elices M, et al. Ayahuasca: Pharmacology, neuroscience and therapeutic potential. *Brain Res Bull.* 2016;126(Pt 1):89-101.

[42] Hanssen MM, Peters ML, Vlaeyen JW, Meevissen YM, Vancleef
      LM. Optimism lowers pain: evidence of the causal status and under-
      lying mechanisms. *Pain.* 2013 Jan;154(1):53-8. doi: 10.1016/j.
      pain.2012.08.006. Epub 2012 Oct 18.

[43] Hobfoll, Stevan E. *Tribalism: The Evolutionary Origins of Fear Politics.*
      Palgrave Macmillan; 1st ed. 2018 Edition, 210pgs.

[44] Hall ET. A System for the Notation of Proxemic Behavior. *American
      Anthropologist.* October 1963;65(5):1003-1026. Doi:10.1525/aa.
      1963.65.5.02a00020

[45] Mensen A, Poryazova R, Schwartz S, Khatami R. Humor as a reward
      mechanism: event-related potentials in the healthy and diseased
      brain. *PLoS One.* 2014 Jan 29;9(1):e85978. doi: 10.1371/journal.
      pone.0085978. eCollection 2014.

[46] Berns GS. Something funny happened to reward. *Trends Cogn Sci.*
      2004 May;8(5):193-4.

[47] Mobbs D, Greicius MD, Abdel-Azim E, Menon V, Reiss AL.
      Humor modulates the mesolimbic reward centers. *Neuron.* 2003 Dec
      4;40(5):1041-8.

[48] Lee C[1], Fernandes MA[2]. Emotional Encoding Context Leads to
      Memory Bias in Individuals with High Anxiety. *Brain Sci.* 2017 Dec
      27;8(1). pii: E6. doi: 10.3390/brainsci8010006.

[49] Aron, E. *The Highly Sensitive Person.* New York, Carol, 1996.

[50] Haberkamp A, Schmidt F, Schmidt T. Rapid visuomotor process-
      ing of phobic images in spider- and snake-fearful participants.
      Acta Psychol (Amst). 2013 Oct;144(2):232-42. doi: 10.1016/j.
      actpsy.2013.07.001. Epub 2013 Aug 7.

[51] Osório C, Probert T, Jones E, Young AH, Robbins I.
      Adapting to Stress: Understanding the Neurobiology of
      Resilience. *Behav Med.* 2017 Oct-Dec;43(4):307-322. doi:
      10.1080/08964289.2016.1170661. Epub 2016 Apr 21.

[52] Sweller, J. (1988) Cognitive Load during Problem Solving: Effects on

Learning. *Cognitive Science,* 12, 257-285. https://doi.org/10.1207/ s15516709cog1202_4

53 Jesse J. Langille. Remembering to Forget: A Dual Role for Sleep Oscillations in Memory Consolidation and Forgetting. *Front Cell Neurosci.* 2019; 13: 71. Published online 2019 Mar 12. doi: 10.3389/fncel.2019.00071. PMCID: PMC6425990. PMID: 30930746

54 Amster LE, Krauss HH. The relationship between life crises and mental deterioration in old age. *Int J Aging Hum Dev* 1974; 5:51-5

55 Johansson L, Guo X, Waern M, Ostling S, Gustafson D, Bengts- son C, Skoog I. Midlife psychological stress and risk of dementia: a 35-year longitudinal population study. *Brain.* 2010:133;2217-2224. Doi:10.1093/brain/awq116

56 Zhang, B., Ma, S., Rachmin, I. *et al.* Hyperactivation of sympathetic nerves drives depletion of melanocyte stem cells. *Nature* (2020). https://doi.org/10.1038/s41586-020-1935-3

57 Hicks E, Hicks J. *The Law of Attraction.* Carlsbad, CA: Hay House, 2006

58 Sullivan M, Tanzer M, Reardon G, Amirault D, Dunbar M, Stan- ish W. The role of presurgical expectancies in predicting pain and function one year following total knee arthroplasty. *Pain.* 2011 Oct;152(10):2287-93. doi: 10.1016/j.pain.2011.06.014. Epub 2011 Jul 18.

59 Hanssen MM, Peters ML, Vlaeyen JW, Meevissen YM, Vancleef LM. Optimism lowers pain: evidence of the causal status and under- lying mechanisms. *Pain.* 2013 Jan;154(1):53-8. doi: 10.1016/j. pain.2012.08.006. Epub 2012 Oct 18.

60 Seebach CL, Kirkhart M, Lating JM, Wegener ST, Song Y, Riley LH 3rd, Archer KR. Examining the role of positive and negative affect in recovery from spine surgery. *Pain.* 2012 Mar;153(3):518-25. doi: 10.1016/j.pain.2011.10.012. Epub 2011 Nov 25.

[61] Byrne, R. *The Secret*. New York : Atria Books ; Hillsboro, OR : Beyond Words Pub., 2006

[62] Merriam-Webster's Collegiate Dictionary (11th ed). Springfield, MA: Merriam-Webster; 2005

[63] Norman KJ, Seiden JA, Klickstein JA, Han X, Hwa LS, DeBold JF, Miczek KA. Social stress and escalated drug self-administration in mice I. Alcohol and corticosterone. *Psychopharmacology (Berl)*. 2015 Mar;232(6):991-1001. doi: 10.1007/s00213-014-3733-9. Epub 2014 Sep 23.

[64] Klanecky Earl AK, Tuliao AP, Landoy BVN, McChargue DE. The Desire to Dissociate Scale: factor analysis, cross-cultural findings, and links to substance-induced dissociation. *Am J Drug Alcohol Abuse*. 2019 Oct 17:1-11. doi: 10.1080/00952990.2019.1669627. [Epub ahead of print]

[65] Dirven BCJ, Homberg JR, Kozicz T, Henckens MJAG. Epigenetic programming of the neuroendocrine stress response by adult life stress. *J Mol Endocrinol*. 2017 Jul;59(1):R11-R31. doi: 10.1530/JME-17-0019. Epub 2017 Apr 11;

Epel, E. S., Blackburn, E. H., Lin, J., Dhabhar, F. S., Adler, N. E., Morrow, J. D., & Cawthon, R. M. (2004). Accelerated telomere shortening in response to life stress. *Proceedings of the National Academy of Sciences of the United States of America, 101*(49), 17312–17315. https://doi.org/10.1073/pnas.0407162101

[66] Daskalakis NP, Rijal CM, King C, Huckins LM, Ressler KJ. Recent Genetics and Epigenetics Approaches to PTSD. *Curr Psychiatry Rep*. 2018 Apr 5;20(5):30. doi: 10.1007/s11920-018-0898-7.

[67] Perrine SA, Eagle AL, George SA, Mulo K, Kohler RJ, Gerard J, Harutyunyan A, Hool SM, Susick LL, Schneider BL, Ghoddoussi F, Galloway MP, Liberzon I, Conti AC. Severe, multimodal stress exposure induces PTSD-like characteristics in a mouse model of single prolonged stress. *Behav Brain Res*. 2016 Apr 15;303:228-37. doi:

10.1016/j.bbr.2016.01.056. Epub 2016 Jan 25.

[68] Omalu B. Chronic traumatic encephalopathy. *Prog Neurol Surg.* 2014;28:38-49. doi: 10.1159/000358761. Epub 2014 Jun 6.

[69] Williams MT. Psychology Cannot Afford to Ignore the Many Harms Caused by Microaggressions. *Perspect Psychol Sci.* 2020 Jan;15(1):38-43. doi: 10.1177/1745691619893362. Epub 2019 Dec 4. PMID: 31801042;

O'Keefe V, Greenfield B. Experiences of Microaggressions Among American Indian and Alaska Native Students in Two Post-Secondary Contexts. *Am Indian Alsk Native Ment Health Res.* 2019;26(3):58-78. doi: 10.5820/aian.2603.2019.58. PMID: 31743415;

Miller LR, Peck BM. A Prospective Examination of Racial Microaggressions in the Medical Encounter. *J Racial Ethn Health Disparities.* 2019 Dec 16. doi: 10.1007/s40615-019-00680-y. [Epub ahead of print] PMID: 31845288

[70] Milkman H. Remedies for alcoholism and substance abuse; an overview. *Drug Alcohol Rev.* 1991;10(1):63-74.

[71] Milkman H, Frosch W. On the preferential abuse of heroine and amphetamine. *Journal of Nervous & Mental Disease.* 156(4):242-248, April 1973.

[72] Rolf Loeber and Jeffrey D. Burke. Developmental Pathways in Juvenile Externalizing and Internalizing Problems *J Res Adolesc.* 2011 Mar; 21(1): 34–46. Published online 2011 Feb 15. doi: 10.1111/j.1532-7795.2010.00713.x. PMCID: PMC3314340. NIHMSID: NIHMS256854. PMID: 22468115

[73] Iacono WG, Malone SM, McGue M. Behavioral disinhibition and the development of early-onset addiction: common and specific influences. *Annu Rev Clin Psychol. 2008; 4():325-48.*

[74] Young Emma. Iceland knows how to stop teen substance abuse but the rest of the world isn't listening. *Mosaic Science,* Jan 16, 2017

[75] Bodhi, Bhikkhu. *The Connected Discourses of the Buddha: A New*

Translation of the Samyutta Nikaya (The Teachings of the Buddha). (2nd Ed), New York: Wisdom Publications; 2005

[76] Morelli T, Agler CS, Divaris K. Genomics of periodontal disease and tooth morbidity. *Periodontol 2000.* 2020 Feb;82(1):143-156. doi: 10.1111/prd.12320. Review. PMID: 31850632

[77] *The Social Dilemma.* Directed by Jeff Orlowski. Written by Jeff Orlowski, Davis Coombe, and Vickie Curtis. Produced by Larissa Rhodes, Exposure Labs, Argent Pictures, The Space Program, 2020

[78] Volkow ND, Fowler JS, Wang GJ, Swanson JM. Dopamine in drug abuse and addiction: results from imaging studies and treatment implications. *Mol Psychiatry.* 2004 Jun;9(6):557-69.

[79] Robins LN, Helzer JE, Davis DH. Narcotic use in southeast Asia and afterward. An interview study of 898 Vietnam returnees. *Arch Gen Psychiatry.* 1975 Aug;32(8):955-61.

[80] Lindgren E, Gray K, Miller G, Tyler R, Wiers CE, Volkow ND, Wang GJ. Food addiction: A common neurobiological mechanism with drug abuse. *Front Biosci (Landmark Ed).* 2018 Jan 1;23:811-836.

[81] Adiv A. Johnson, Kemal Akman, Stuart R.G. Calimport, Daniel Wuttke, Alexandra Stolzing, and João Pedro de Magalhães. The Role of DNA Methylation in Aging, Rejuvenation, and Age-Related Disease. *Rejuvenation Res.* 2012 Oct; 15(5): 483–494. doi: 10.1089/rej.2012.1324. PMCID: PMC3482848. PMID: 23098078

[82] Wimmer ME, Briand LA, Fant B, Guercio LA, Arreola AC, Schmidt HD, Sidoli S, Han Y, Garcia BA, Pierce RC. Paternal cocaine taking elicits epigenetic remodeling and memory deficits in male progeny. *Mol Psychiatry.* 2017 Nov;22(11):1653. doi: 10.1038/mp.2017.71. Epub 2017 Mar 21.

[83] O'Dair B. Compulsion without the Chemicals. Time Magazine Special Edition: The Science of Addiction. Meredith Corp. 2019

[84] Newton, Casey. Everything you need to know about Section 230:

The most important law for online speech *The Verge,* theverge.com, Mar. 3, 2020

[85] Garcia R. Neurobiology of fear and specific phobias. *Learn Mem.* 2017 Aug 16;24(9):462-471. doi: 10.1101/lm.044115.116. Print 2017 Sep.

[86] Griffin L, Youssef NA. Phobia with hallucinations and PTSD: Can amygdala dysfunction be a common unified lesion in the RDoC sense? *Ann Clin Psychiatry.* 2017 Aug;29(3):207-208.

[87] Byrne SP, Rapee RM, Richardson R, Malhi GS, Jones M, Hudson JL. D-cycloserine enhances generalization of fear extinction in children. *Depress Anxiety.* 2015 Jun;32(6):408-14. doi: 10.1002/da.22356. Epub 2015 Mar 10.

[88] Agness L. *Change Your Life with NLP: The Powerful Way to Make Your Whole Life Better with Neuro-Linguistic Programming.* New York, NY. Skyhorse Publishing 2013

[89] Michael James Winkelman *Shamanism: A biopsychosocial paradigm of consciousness and healing.* 2nd Ed. Santa Barbara, CA: ABC-CLIO, 2010. ISBN: 978-0-313-38181-2

[90] Tommy K Begay, Michael A Grandner. Sleep and cardiometabolic health in indigenous populations: importance of socio-cultural context. *Sleep Med.* 2019 Jul;59:88-89. doi: 10.1016/j.sleep.2018.11.013. Epub 2018 Nov 29.

[91] Nacoti M, Ciocca A, Giupponi A, Brambillasca, P, Lussana F, Pisano M, Goisis G, Bonacina D, Fazzi F, Naspro R, Longhi L, Cereda M, Montaguti C. At the Epicenter of the Covid-19 Pandemic and Humanitarian Crises in Italy: Changing Perspectives on Preparation and Mitigation. *New England Journal of Medicine Catalyst.* 2020 March-April, Mar 21;1(2)1-5. Doi:10.1056/CAT.20.0080

ABOUT THE AUTHOR

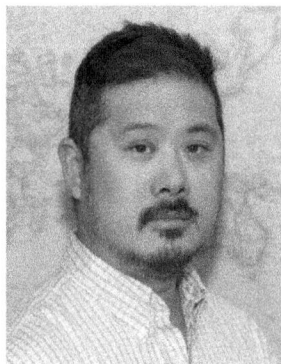

KARL CHING grew up traveling between the small towns connected by dusty two laned roads of the American West. A graduate of the University of California at Berkeley and the UCLA School of Dentistry, he has nurtured a keen interest in healing and traditional medicines for over 30 years. In a quest to find the meaning of true healing, he has delved into the age-old knowledge of generations to find key elements missing in modern medicine. Empowering modern-day health care professionals, counselors, clergy, mentors, and potential patients alike, he reimagines a future that nurtures both broken bodies and ailing souls with the intangible skills learned through a millennium. When not seeing patients, Karl enjoys reveling in nature, strumming his guitar, and contemplating on his blog www.healing-reimagined.com.